CONTENTS

Introduction

Intermittent fasting is a very natural way of structuring our eating. Before we had a constant supply of food on demand, fasting was the norm, and it is still a very natural process for many animals, some of which don't eat for weeks or months at a time while hibernating. Our hunter-gatherer ancestors, after all, did not have the luxury of constant access to food, so fasting was not really a choice for them, but they survived some seriously difficult conditions all the same.

Our energy requirements are, of course, very different today than they were during the age that we had to hunt our own food. At that time, we needed bursts of energy in order to overcome situations that occasionally cropped up. Today, our energy requirements are more sustained, so it stands to reason that we would not fast for extended periods.

In explaining what intermittent fasting is, it is perhaps pertinent to explain what it is not. Intermittent fasting is not a free ticket to binge on everything your eyes see as long as you 'starve' yourself within the required period. Anyone approaching intermittent fasting from such a standpoint is doing themselves more harm than good. The basics of good nutrition, lean proteins, plenty of fresh fruit and vegetables, good sources of fiber, and good fats do not change because you are structuring the times at which you eat. If you wish to see all of the benefits that intermittent fasting can offer, then maintaining good nutrition with the occasional treat is imperative. Intermittent fasting has nothing to do with starving yourself. The term 'starvation' implies that you do not have access to food and that you are, in some way, experiencing negative health effects from not eating. Starvation is generally not deliberate or controlled. Instead, intermittent fasting means that although you do have access to food, you choose when to eat and the experience is not damaging to your health in the way that starvation would be. Intermittent fasting involves assigning a pattern for eating around specific times.

You may be wondering how that is any different from eating breakfast, lunch, and dinner at specific times. If you consider the fact that you usually don't eat meals at specific times but rather when and if you are hungry, that shows a distinct difference between the two ideas. When you practice intermittent fasting, you structure your day in fasting hours and eating hours.

It does take a mindset change to introduce intermittent fasting as a lifestyle since you have likely grown up with the idea that having three square meals per day is the healthiest way to eat. We have also had phrases like "breakfast is the most important meal of the day" drummed into our heads, which is usually just a marketing tool for sugar-filled cereal brands.

An intermittent fasting lifestyle has a huge number of health benefits including weight loss, fat burning, stabilization of blood sugar, limiting of disease, increased rate of cell repair, and increased longevity.

Remember: Intermittent fasting isn't for everybody. It's not something that everybody needs to do. It's simply an instrument that can be valuable for certain individuals.

Once you've made up your mind to attempt intermittent fasting, always bear in mind that you have to eat well too. It's unrealistic to gorge on food during the eating time frames and hope to get more fit and improve in wellbeing.

Chapter 1:The Basics of Intermittent Fasting

What is Intermittent Fasting?

Intermittent fasting is a regimen of controlled meal placement and controlled periods of fasting. At first glance, it may simply look like meal skipping, but the added element that can't be missed or forgotten is ensuring that our bodies are getting the nourishment they require throughout each day, even on the days when we've chosen not to eat anything. The core concept of intermittent fasting doesn't dictate what you should or should not be eating, but it does dictate the intervals at which you eat and at which you fast.

With intermittent fasting, you're cutting down your calorie intake by shaving off a meal here and there throughout your week and you're giving your body the chance to adapt and boost its hormone production that will allow you to access and break down those stores of fat your body has created over the years. By doing this, you'll find that your body is creating energy, even when you have not eaten recently. Because your body will be getting accustomed to this method of living and this means of procuring energy, you'll find that you have more energy on a more consistent basis throughout the day. Because your body has onboard stores of energy that it can now access, you won't experience those midday slumps or crashes. You won't feel faint after several hours of not eating, because your body is still getting everything it needs from those stores!

Benefits of Intermittent Fasting on Women

Reduction constant worry and inflammation

Intermittent fasting lowers stress, which is among the most risky methods of fast aging and also other chronic illnesses. Molecules line proteins and DNA react with free radicals, and get destroyed. Intermittent fasting, therefore, is important in fighting inflammation in the body and destroying any molecules that bring worries constantly.

Intermittent fasting has been found to lower inflammation. As you know, inflammation causes a lot of many chronic diseases such as diabetes, dementia, Alzheimer's disease, obesity, and much more. Now, there are many ways that intermittent fasting helps you get rid of inflammation. The first one being autophagy, as you know, intermittent fasting aids in cell rejuvenation where it eats out the old cells and rejuvenating them with the newer ones which are stronger. If your body does not rejuvenate itself with more new cells, inflammation can be caused by the older ones that have stayed for an extended period.

As you know, the average diet does not allow for cell rejuvenation to happen; this is where intermittent fasting comes in as it has been proven to help with the process of autophagy. Another way intermittent fasting enables you to get rid of inflammation would be by producing ketones. When you are fasting, your body uses up all the glycogen stores, which makes it start using stored fat for fuel, and when fats are broken down for energy, ketones are produced. One of the most popular ketones in your body will block a part of your immune system, which is responsible for inflammatory disorders. Another way intermittent fasting helps you lower the risk of inflammation is by making you insulin sensitive. When your body becomes insulin resistant, you will be holding much glucose in your bloodstream. More glucose in your blood will create inflammation, and intermittent fasting allows your body to get rid of all the glucose, which helps you reduce inflammation in your body.

Reducing gut problem

Since humans are almost constantly eating, the digestive system is always working. With all the food consumed, including processed food, this may lead to gut-related problems. That is why Intermittent fasting is like giving your digestive system a day off from all the work it has to do. You're allowing it to rest and be cleansed of impurities. Think about it. Your digestive system is constantly at work trying to maintain homeostasis in your body, and if you eat every single day, it never gets a break. Your body will thank you for finally listening to it and allowing it to recharge. Your body has this sort of innate intelligence to heal itself if you allow the process to happen, and intermittent fasting is a key to this. Keep track of your digestion before and after doing a fast, and see how you feel physically. Write down how you feel if you want to feel and see a difference.

Weight-Loss and belly fats

Most people practice intermittent fasting as way of losing weight as you only in a few meals taken. It improves your metabolic rate, and this is important in burning extra fats in the body including belly fats. Research has shown that a person loses 3-8% of their weight if the do intermittent fasting for 3-24 weeks. During this period, 4-7% of the people in the study lost belly fats which is usually very toxic and may cause illnesses.

Healthy Heart

Intermittent fasting keeps the heart healthy by preventing heart diseases. It controls the sugar levels in the body thereby preventing high cholesterol levels, inflammatory markers, and high blood pressure. This keeps your heart healthy.

Low Diabetes risk

Intermittent fasting helps in reducing the insulin levels in the body and this helps in lowering the type 2 diabetes risk which is an illness that is common. The characteristics of diabetes include the blood sugar levels that are high if you are battling insulin. Therefore, intermittent fasting lowers the insulin levels and thus helps in preventing this particular illness. It as well helps in protecting the damages that may affect the kidneys.

Prevention of Polycystic ovary syndrome (PCOS)

PCOS is a hormonal disorder that affects women in the reproductive age. Intermittent fasting has been found to lower insulin levels in people with PCOS drastically.

Autophagy

It is the process through which the body starts the "waste elimination" procedures. Cells in the body break down and metabolize the dysfunctional proteins piling in the cells of the body. The autophagy process protects you from ailments like Alzheimer's disease, which has no cure.

Cancer prevention

Your body becomes risk-free from any cancer risks when the dysfunctional cells that pile up in your body over time are eliminated. Among the features of cancer is uncontrolled cell growth; inter mitten fasting controls the metabolic rate of the body and in the process lowers the risk of cancer.Intermittent fasting also reduces several impacts of chemotherapy.

Brain health

Since intermittent fasting is better for your body, then it is best for your brain. Reduction of oxidative stress and various worries is advantageous for your brain fitness. Recurrent fasting increases the development of new nerves, which improves the functioning of your brain. It also helps in increasing brain hormone levels known as the Brain-derived neurotrophic factors, which helps fight depression and any other brain-related illnesses. Intermittent fasting also helps fight brain damages caused by stroke.

Improved health in Perimenopausal women:

Intermittent fasting has been found to lower perimenopausal women's health risks such as blood sugar balance and insulin sensitivity.

Increased lifespan

Intermittent fasting can help you live longer due to its ability to control metabolism rates, regulating blood sugar levels, and eliminating any dysfunctional cells within your body.

Improved Immunity

Fasting and calorie restriction without pushing the body into a malnourished state has been said to be among the most potent physiological interventions to improve the immunity of the body.

In a study done on rodents in regards to intermittent fasting and mammary tumors, the rodents experienced a 40-80 percent reduction in tumor incidences. That is a drastic difference!

Another theory states that cancer cells are not protected by the same protective signals that are stimulated when the body is fasting. The rest of the body is on lockdown, but the cancer cells are still 'exposed,' giving the immune system and white blood cells a chance to attack and fight the cancer cells more effectively as well as improving the results of cancer treatments. This protective state can also help in protecting mammalian cells and human cells, from the destructive toxins in the chemotherapy.

It is said that fasting can help regenerate a stronger immune system. If harsher treatments have already depleted the immune system, intermittent fasting can assist in rebuilding that system to continue to combat the cancerous cells.

Improvement in Fertility

Doctors who specialize in IVF treatments give a positive report about intermittent fasting. It has been noted that fasting has helped the couples who were struggling to conceive even through in vitro fertilization, or on synthetic contraception.

Whenever IVF specialized doctors find a patient who is struggling to conceive, the first thing they do is analyze their diet. The amount of nutrition and calories a person consumes affects their chances of getting pregnant. Some people are even asked to take up intermittent fasting to achieve an ideal body mass index.

Gynecologists have noticed that fasting has significant benefits in increasing a woman's fertility. This happens due to the many changes that her body goes through while fasting. Intermittent fasting plays a direct role in improving fertility by:

- Pulling out excess and synthetic hormones
- Cleansing the liver
- Alkalizing the bloodstream
- Rebooting the natural hormone process of the body
- Flushing out the unwanted toxins
- Helping women to attain the right BMI
- Decreasing inflammation
- Balancing blood sugar levels
- Boosting metabolism and immune system
- Getting the reproductive system ready

Disadvantages of Intermittent Fasting for Women over 50

Getting Started Takes an Adjustment

Any lifestyle change takes an adjustment, and it can take months for something to become a habit. Naturally, intermittent fasting is quite an adjustment for people who are used to grazing on food throughout the day. This means that if you push yourself to go into an advanced version of intermittent fasting when you first begin, you can become overwhelmed. But if you start slowly and allow your body to adjust in its own time, you will find it happens much more naturally and becomes easy to stick to.

You do not have to deny yourself food when you are hungry and suffer through hunger pangs. Instead, practice fasting when you are naturally satisfied and eat when you are hungry. If you slowly increase the length of your fasting window, your body will adjust without difficulty, and before long, your body will discover the eating and fasting windows that the human body is naturally inclined to.

Potential to Overeat

While intermittent fasting should naturally reduce caloric intake, if a person pushes themselves to fast when they are overly hungry, it might lead to overeating during their eating window. This is because the person feels hungry for so long when fasting when they can finally eat their body believes it must make up for the calories it missed. The result is that the person either hits a weight loss plateau or even experience increased weight.

Thankfully, this is easy to avoid. If you listen to your body by eating when you are hungry and fasting when you are satisfied, you shouldn't overeat. By practicing eating mindfully and slowly, you can also avoid overeating, and you will become more attuned to your body and know when you have eaten enough and can stop.

Possible Leptin Imbalance

The hormone leptin is important as it signals to your body that you are full have no longer need to eat. But when a person practices intermittent fasting, it may temporarily disrupt this hormone's production. However, this is usually only a short-term problem, and once a person's body adjusts to their fasting and eating windows, their leptin will balance itself out.

Typically, a leptin imbalance is only a real problem when a person dives head-first into intermittent fasting and attempt to practice advanced level fasting when they are still only a beginner.

You May Become Dehydrated

Many people do not drink enough water. In general, doctors recommend that we drink water, half of our body's weight in pounds.

Not only do many people not drink enough water as it is, but this can make dehydration worse when a person is practicing fasting. This is because fasting boosts the metabolism, and when your cells are in a metabolic accelerated state, they require more water for fuel. If you are not giving them enough water during periods of fasting, you can quickly become dehydrated. Not only that but when fasting, you are likely to lose a lot of water weight, which can result in dehydration and a deficiency in electrolytes. Make sure that you not only drink plenty of water but also consume enough electrolytes to prevent this. Thankfully, dehydration is easy to avoid if you remain proactive.

Not Everyone Can Practice Intermittent Fasting

Intermittent fasting is a beautiful and healthy lifestyle for the general population. After all, the human body is designed for practice periods of fasting naturally. However, not every person can practice fasting. Some people, due to chronic illness, may be unable to participate. Ultimately, you must ask your doctor if you are healthy enough to practice short-term fasting.

For instance, people with severe diabetes, metabolic disorders, or those who are pregnant may be unable to practice fasting, even short-term. Whenever you are making a lifestyle change, it is essential first to discuss the matter with your doctor to determine if it is a healthy choice for you individually.

How intermittent fasting works

When you eat, your food is converted into sugar that serves as your body's fuel and is stored in the liver. As you eat, your insulin levels increase to help the body store this influx of energy. However, your liver can only store so much, and it is a limited amount, before it reaches capacity. Your body fat serves as this backup storage so when your liver is full, the excess energy is stored as body fat. Although energy stored in the liver is accessible, body fat has unlimited storage capacity.

Eating gives your body a lot of work to do – breaking down food particles, digesting, and extracting energy and nutrients. The periods when you are not eating, your body turns to the stored energy to fuel your activities and keep you going.

What this means is that when you are fasting, there is a significant absence of energy coming from meals. Within hours, energy from your liver is depleted, and your insulin level drops. Your body senses this change and turns to the backup storage to begin using stored energy in the form of body fat. In other words, fasting helps your body burn fat. Essentially, you are either accumulating energy by eating or burning up energy when you are not. The key to maintaining a healthy weight and generally staying healthy is to strike a balance between storing and using energy.

Your body does not need you to feed it frequently for it to have enough energy. If you are a normal healthy person, your body already has enough energy to last you longer than you realize. If you don't give your body time to use its stored energy, it can result in being overweight. The reason for storing energy in the first place is so that it can be used later. How can it be used if you don't allow your body a break from accumulating it? If you were meant to eat continuously, there would be no need for anything in place to reserve it.

On the other hand, staying away from food for too long can have adverse effects on your body. As much as you don't want to be overweight, being underweight is never healthy, and why you need to find a balance between eating and not eating. A good way to do that is by introducing a pattern of eating that helps you to reduce the number of hours you eat (without necessarily focusing on reducing calories). When you reduce your eating hours, your calorie intake declines.

Chapter 2: The Science of Intermittent Fasting

Reduce, reuse, and recycle is a popular phrase you're likely to hear in discussions relating to environmental sustainability. This is similar in many ways to what autophagy does – reducing or breaking down and repairing parts of your cells, and then recycling important body chemicals that can be reused by the liver.

Autophagy is the natural process that removes toxic materials and broken cells from your body to create new and healthier cells. The term comes from Latin which translates to self-eating (auto= "self" and phagy= "to eat"). In a weird way, this means your body is eating itself! Don't panic, it's a good thing. It's a rejuvenation process for your body.

If you fully realize what autophagy is and how to make it work for you, you will be quick to find ways to consciously stimulate the process because it can keep you feeling and looking younger than your real age! Older adults, in particular, can use this natural process to increase longevity.

Here's a simple analogy of how autophagy works that I think a lot of women can relate to. Think of what happens inside your kitchen when you are preparing a delicious meal. You are creating something heartfelt and necessary while at the same time making a mess and producing waste. If you leave your kitchen dirty after preparing your meal, it will be difficult to make your next meal. So, you do what any self-respecting woman does: throw or put away leftovers, clean the counter, put away unused ingredients, and recycle some of the food if you can. This is exactly how autophagy works in your body. It cleans up after you!

A big mess is created each day inside the body. This mess includes parts of dead cells, damaged proteins, and harmful particles that prevent optimal body function. When you were much younger, the process of autophagy clears this mess up as quickly as possible, keeping them looking young and supple. But as you grow older, the cleanup process slows down. Dirt, mess, and crumbs start to build up internally due to old age. If left unattended, the buildup can result in rapid aging, increased risk of cancer and dementia, as well as other diseases associated with old age.

But growing older doesn't mean you're doomed to have an inefficient cellular cleaning process. You can stimulate the process of autophagy and make it work as it used to when you were a lot younger. An effective way to do that is by doing something that induces stress such as decreasing insulin levels and increasing your glucagon levels. In simpler terms, go without food for longer than you usually would. When you get really hungry as you do when you fast, your glucagon is increased and stimulates autophagy.

You can achieve some positive life-altering benefits by simply activating autophagy. But before going into the immense health benefits, let us consider the science behind the process, albeit briefly.

How Does Autophagy Work?

The process of autophagy involves small "hunter" particles that go around your body, looking for cells or cell components that are old and damaged. The hunter particles then take these cell components apart, getting rid of the damaged parts and saving the useful parts to make new cells later. These hunter cells can also use useful leftover parts to create energy for the body.

Autophagy has been found to happen in all organisms that are multi-cellular, like animals and plants, in addition to humans. While the study of these larger organisms and how autophagy works in their cells is lesser-known, more studies are being done on humans and how changes in diet can affect their body's autophagy.

The other function that autophagy serves is that it helps cells to carry out their death when it is time for them to die. There are times when cells are programmed to die because of a number of different factors. Sometimes these cells need assistance in their death, and autophagy can help them with this or can help to clean up after their death. The human body is all about life and death, and these processes are continually going on without our knowledge to keep us healthy and in good form.

The process of autophagy has been going on inside of us for many, many years, since the beginning of humans. This process has been kept around inside of our bodies because of the multitude of benefits it can provide us with. It is also essential for the health of our bodies, as being able to get rid of waste and damaged parts that are no longer useful to us is essential to our health. If we were unable to get rid of damaged or broken cells, these damaged particles would build up and eventually make us sick. Our bodies are extremely efficient in everything that they do, and waste disposal is no different.

More about autophagy and its relation to energy production is being studied in recent years, as this topic is of interest to humans. Autophagy can use old cell parts and recycle them to create new energy that the organism (like the human or animal) can then use to do its regular functions like walking and breathing. Now, people are studying what happens when humans rely on this form of energy production instead of the energy they would get from ingesting food throughout the day. This is where autophagy and Intermittent fasting come together. We will look at how they work together throughout the rest of this book as we delve deeply into intermittent fasting and autophagy and how they work together to allow for things like weight loss or disease prevention.

The Benefits of autophagy

Some people are said to have different biological and chronological age. That is to say, their age is different from their quality of their life. Women are more likely to worry about showing signs of aging or looking older than men. Thankfully, you can look younger by activating autophagy. What the process does to your cells is to remove toxins and recycle cells instead of creating new ones. These rejuvenated cells will behave like new and work better.

Your skin is constantly exposed to harmful lights, air, chemicals, as well as harsh weather conditions. This causes damage to your skin cells. As the damaged cells continue to accumulate, your skin begins to wrinkle, lose elasticity, and no longer appear smooth. The process of autophagy repairs your skin cells that might have been partly damaged to make your skin glow and healthier. In the same way that wear and tear happens with things you use frequently, wear and tear (microtear) also happens to your muscles as you use them especially during exercises. Your muscles become inflamed and require repairs. What this means is you need more energy to use these specific muscles. The process of autophagy in your cells will degrade the damaged parts in the muscle, reduce the amount of energy sent to the muscle, and ensure energy balance.

To keep your metabolism working well, your cells need to be in top shape. The powerhouse of your cell is the mitochondria. A lot of harmful trash is left behind in the mitochondria as it performs its function of burning fat and making adenosine triphosphate (ATP) – the molecule that stores all the energy you need to do almost everything. This harmful trash can damage your cells. Autophagy ensures that these toxins are promptly taken care of to prevent damage to your cells and keep them in a healthy state.

Several processes and activities that occur during your cellular cleaning and repairs also help you to maintain a healthy weight. For example, when toxins are removed from your cells through autophagy and you successfully excrete them, your fat cells can no longer store these toxins. Also, when you fast for short periods (12 to 16 hours), autophagy is activated, fat-burning also takes place, and since it is not a prolonged fast, your proteins are spared. All these activities and processes help to make you leaner and fitter.

The cells of your gastrointestinal tract hardly ever take breaks. You put them to work consistently, and this can affect digestive health. Autophagy helps repair and restore the cells. When you stop eating for long periods you give your gut ample time to rest and heal. Giving your gut some rest (from digesting your meal) is vital for an overall improved digestive health.

Certain neurodegenerative diseases such as Parkinson's disease and Alzheimer's disease are a result of too much accumulation of damaged proteins around the brain cells. Autophagy clears this clutter of damaged proteins that don't work as they should. Dementia is not a normal part of aging, even though it is largely linked to older people. You can prevent all these diseases by activating autophagy. If your brain cells are clear of clutter (damaged protein cells), you will perform cognitive functions optimally.

Using Intermittent Fasting to Induce Autophagy

Autophagy functions in the following way. When a decrease in nutrients is noticed within a cell, this decrease in nutrients acts as a signal for the cell to create small pockets within a membrane (a thin barrier layer) that are called autophagosomes. These small pockets (autophagosomes) move through the cell and find debris and damaged particles floating around within the cell. The small pockets then consume this debris by absorbing it into its inner space. The debris is then enclosed in the membrane (the thin barrier layer) and is moved to a place in the cell called the Lysosome. A lysosome is a part of a cell that acts as a center for degradation, breakdown, or disassembly. This part of the cell gets debris and damaged cell parts delivered to it by the autophagosomes. Once these damaged cell parts are delivered, the lysosomes then break them down. By breaking them down, these parts can be recycled and used for energy.

The most common way to induce autophagy in a person is by way of starvation. This is not to say that a person must starve themselves, but that they starve their cells of nutrition temporarily. This is why people turn to fasting in order to induce autophagy. Low nutrition levels within the cells is the most common way that autophagy is triggered, as it is a process that creates energy within the cell. By knowing this, scientists have concluded that by inducing starvation within the cells, one can intentionally upregulate autophagy in their body. Intermittent Fasting involves periods of fasting, which then induces a state of starvation within the cells (simply meaning that there is no energy being consumed to use for energy) and so it induces autophagy in the cells to make energy.

Other Ways to activate Autophagy

One of the quickest ways to activate autophagy is by staying away from food for longer periods. In other words, intermittent fasting can create just the right level of stress on your body to kick start the internal cleanup process. Going without food leads to an energy deficit, and that induces autophagy ridding your body of decaying cells and accumulated junk. So, besides the widely known weight loss benefits of intermittent fasting, perhaps a far-reaching positive aspect of practicing intermittent fasting is activating autophagy.

Starvation

The most common way to induce autophagy in a person is by way of starvation. Autophagy is triggered by a decrease in nutrients within a cell. As I mentioned above, this decrease in nutrients acts as a signal within the cell to begin the process of autophagy, which is exactly how Intermittent Fasting works.

Aerobic Exercise

One other way to activate autophagy is through exercise. Aerobic exercise has been shown through studies to increase autophagy in the cells of the muscles, the heart, the brain, lungs, pancreas and the liver. This is particularly true for areas of the body where the process of metabolic regulation occurs.

Sleep

Sleep is very important for autophagy. If you have ever gone a few days without a proper, restful sleep, you know that you begin to feel a decline in your mental abilities rather quickly. This could be because of your brain's decreased autophagy functioning. The number of hours that you are in bed does not matter if the sleep is not good quality, though. Quality sleep for the right hours is what is needed to maintain good brain function and keep your brain's autophagy going.

Specific Foods

The consumption of specific foods has been shown to induce or promote autophagy. We will look at some examples of these foods later on in this book. The added benefit is that not only do they trigger autophagy in the cells of your body, these foods are also shown to have numerous other health benefits.

Chapter 3:Types of Intermittent fasting for Women Over 50

16:8 Method

The 16:8 fasting diet is similar to the 12-hour fast except that it requires a slightly longer fasting window. This fasting diet can be a little more challenging for some people to adapt to as it requires 16 hours of fasting and only 8 hours of eating. This means that in 8 hours, you need to consume any meals and snacks that you want to for the day.

Despite being more intense, the 16:8 diet is still typically an easy one to adjust to. With some minor adjustments to your daily schedule, you can easily accommodate the longer fasting window. Typically, most people who do the 16:8 diet cut out their regular breakfast meal and focus on lunch and dinner instead. This makes it quite a simple adjustment once you get used to skipping breakfast.

The most common way of eating in alignment with this fast is to stop eating at 8 PM each day and then eat again at noon the next day. This is typically the easiest way to accommodate the 16 hours of fasting. However, you can also choose to stop eating after dinner and eat an earlier lunch the next day. How you choose to adjust the fasting window is not nearly as important as making sure that you get the full 16 hours of fasting each day.

For some people, the 16:8 diet may still be quite similar to how they already eat. For both the 12-hour fast and the 16:8 diet, many people find that they instinctively eat this way, to begin with. However, being stricter about not eating during that fasting window can support you in seeing greater health benefits from your dietary habits. When you are eating in alignment with the 16:8 fasting practice, you see even greater improvements similar to what you see from the 12-hour fast. This makes it a great "step-up" for anyone who is not seeing all of the results that they desire to see from the 12-hour fast.

14:10 Method

In this method, you have 14 hours of fasting, followed by a period of 10 hours where you should eat. The difference between this method and the 16:8 is that this method has two more hours of the eating period.

20:4 Method

This method is really intense as it needs a person to fast for 20 hours each day and an eating window of 4. The eating window where one should gain energy and nutrients is quite short. Whereas the 14:10 method was an easier step down from 16:8 method, 20:4 method is absolutely an increase in terms of difficulty. It's a more intense method certainly, for it requires 20 hours of fasting within each day with only a 4-hour eating window for the individual to gain all his or her nutrients and energy.

Fasting, in this manner, does not cause any harm to your body. However, if you are completely new to fasting, using this method may have a dramatic impact on your body, most of which may not be comfortable or pleasant. This is a regimen you will want to approach carefully. It is advisable to be sure-footed in fasting before upping your game to this level. Test the waters with something less stringent before jumping headlong into this regimen.

If you choose to go with this regimen, be sure not to practice this way of eating for an extended period. That is to say, use the 20:4 regimen for short periods. Do not use this method for more than 3 to 4 days consecutively, or at most, for a whole week at a stretch. Always keep in mind that your body system requires time to adjust to new changes.

Eat-Stop-Eat (24-Hour) Method

During this 24-hour window, absolutely no food should be consumed. Individuals are also encouraged to avoid drinking any drinks that may be too high in calories, such as whole milk lattés or smoothies.

This variation of the diet is often called the "eat-stop-eat" diet because it only requires one day of true change every week. Otherwise, you can eat whatever you want and however, you want. For those who are seeking to incorporate weekly dieting into their eating plans, the 24-hour weekly fast is a great place to start. This is a relatively relaxed place to start. For some people, it may offer plenty enough benefits to make it a good place to stay, too. For others, they may prefer to adjust to the 5:2 diet after they get used to it so that they can see greater results from their efforts.

It is important to be cautious of how the 24-hour weekly fast impacts you. While some people find great success with this, other people find that one single day per week is not frequently enough, so their body never fully acclimates. As a result, they end up experiencing headaches, fatigue, or even irritability during their fasting day. For most, these symptoms outweigh the benefits that they gain, which results in them not maintaining the 24-hour fasting cycle. If you still want to give this eating pattern a try, you may benefit from first using the 16:8 fasting method before adjusting to test out the 24-hour weekly fasting. This can support your body by getting used to the changes.

Lean-Gains Method

This method basically focuses on the collective efforts of a healthy diet, fasting, and rigorous exercise. This method is popular because it directly turns fat into muscle. The objective is fast for 14-16 hours within each day.

The best approach towards this method is waking up and fasting up to 1 pm while stretching and doing some warm-ups before midday. After midday, you can do an exercise of choice for up to an hour and end with breaking fast at 1 pm.

12:12 Method

The average person fasts for around eight hours every night. So, the 12-hour fast is not a far stretch from what you likely already naturally do in your everyday life. When you follow the 12-hour fasting diet, you want to maintain equal lengths of fasting and eating windows each day. The easiest way to do this is to eat an earlier supper and a later breakfast.

Completing the 12-hour fast diet should not take too much adjustment to your traditional eating routine. Chances are, you probably already eat pretty close to this type of schedule in your daily life, anyway. The biggest adjustment to this type of fasting is that you truly need to cut out late-night snacking. Late-night snacking tends to be the primary way that people consume food between 7 PM and 7 AM, anyway. Letting go of this habit can support you in taking on the intermittent fasting eating cycles and gaining many benefits without any drastic changes to your routine. Another reason why this diet may be easier for beginners is that you still have plenty of time to consume the same number of calories per day than you are used to. Other diets with shorter eating windows typically do not leave enough time for you to get quite as many calories into your day, which can lead to a bit of a transition phase as you get used to your new eating cycles.

The 12-hour fast is a great practice for those who are just starting out with intermittent fasting. Alternatively, it might be a better consideration for those who cannot commit to a more intense variation of the diet for health reasons. Because it does not require any major changes to your present eating routines, it is easy to adapt to and can support you in maintaining any other dietary requirements that you may need to consider.

Alternate-Day Method

This specific protocol requires that you eat regularly one day and then fast the next day. You are allowed to eat any food that you like on your non-fasting days. This particular protocol can be modified so that you only have 500 calories on your fasting days.

The alternate-day diet is often touted as the most effective form of intermittent fasting in regards to weight loss. Overweight and obese adults who follow this approach have been shown to lose as much as eight percent of their body fat in two months. Middle-aged people, a population that tends to struggle with weight loss particularly, seem to benefit from this program particularly. Much of the fat loss is the dangerous belly fat that can lead to heart disease and inflammation. The weight-loss benefits of the alternate day diet may actually supersede those of traditional calorie-cutting alone.

People who follow the alternate day diet and exercise regularly have been able to lose up to twice as much weight as those who merely cut calories. That figure goes up to as much as six times more weight loss for individuals who follow the alternate day diet and exercise, as opposed to those who only exercise. Again, exercising on fasting days may be difficult, especially at first. You may find that the best plan for you is to exercise twice as much on regular days and either not exercise or exercise a minimal amount on fasting days.

This is the ideal fasting protocol for anyone who desires to lose weight. It is very effective because of the frequent calorie restriction throughout the week. Your eating will only be restricted for half the time. For the rest of the time, you will enjoy your meals normally. On your fast days, you are allowed to have all sorts of beverages, including green tea, coffee, or water. All these should be calorie-free. You can modify this protocol so that you consume only 20 to 25 percent of your daily caloric requirements. This is equivalent to 500 calories per day. Studies show that women prefer this form of calorie restriction because it lasts for only a day, and they get to choose the foods they want to eat the following day. Traditional diets often require deprivation almost every day and restrictions regarding food choice.

Spontaneous Skipping Method

Meal skipping is an extremely flexible form of intermittent fasting that can provide all of the benefits of intermittent fasting but with less of the strict scheduling. If you are not someone who has a typical schedule or who feels as though a stricter variation of the intermittent fasting diet will serve you, meal skipping is a viable alternative.

Many people who choose to use meal skipping find it to be a great way to listen to their bodies and follow their basic instincts. If they are not hungry, they simply don't eat that meal. Instead, they wait for the next one. Meal skipping can also be helpful for people who have time constraints and who may not always be able to get in a certain meal of the day. Often, people discover that they simply don't become hungry 3+ times per day. So, instead of eating several meals, they only eat when they are hungry.

It is important to realize that with meal skipping, you may not always be maintaining a 10-16-hour window of fasting. As a result, you may not get every benefit that comes from other fasting diets. However, this may be a great solution to people who want an intermittent fasting diet that feels more natural to them. It may also be a great idea for those who are looking to begin listening to their body more so that they can adjust to a more intense variation of the diet with greater ease. In other words, it can be a great transitional diet for you if you are not ready to jump into one of the other fasting diets just yet.

Crescendo Method

The method is best suited for females (since their anatomies can be so detrimentally sensitive to high-intensity fasts). Basically, this method is made for gradual additions, gentle introductions, and internal awareness, but it is subject to what works best for you.

In this method, a person begins by fasting for only 2 or 3 days a week, and on days they fast, it's not usually intense. The remaining days of the week are open to eating, but one should try and eat a diet that is healthy during the week.

Chapter 4:What to Eat and What to Avoid

What to eat

Berries.

Berries are very healthy, incredibly flavorful, and much lower in calories and sugar than you might think! Their tart sweetness can really bring a smoothie to life and they make an absolutely delicious snack on their own without any help from things like cream or sugar.

Cruciferous vegetables.

These are the vegetables like cabbage, Brussels sprouts, broccoli, and cauliflower. These are wonderful additions to your diet because they're packed with vital nutrients and with fiber that your body will love and use with a quickness!

Eggs.

Eggs are such a great addition to your diet because they're packed to the gills with protein, you can do just about anything with them, they're easy to prepare, they travel well if you hard boil them, and they can pair with just about anything. They're a great protein source for salads, and they're good on their own as well.

Fish.

Fish are a wonderful source of protein and healthy fats. White fish, in particular, is typically very lean, but fish like salmon that have a little bit of color in them are packed with protein, fats, and oils that are great for you. They're good for brain and heart health, and there's a huge array of delicious things you can do with them.

Healthy starches like certain potatoes (with skins!)

Red potatoes, in particular, are perfectly fine to eat, even if you're trying to lose weight because your body can use those carbs for fuel and the skins are packed with minerals that your body will enjoy. A little bit of potato here and there can-do good things for your nutrition, but they are also a great way to feel like you're getting a little more of those fun foods that you should cut back on.

Legumes.

Beans, beans, the magical fruit. They're packed with protein and the starch in them just makes them stick to your ribs without making you pay for it later. They're wonderful in soups, salads, and just about any other meal of the day that you're looking to fill out. By adding beans to your regimen, you might find that your meals stick with you a little bit longer and leave you feeling more satisfied than you thought possible.

Nuts.

I know you've heard people talking about how a handful of almonds makes a great snack and if you're anything like me, you've always had kind of a hard time believing it. Nuts, as it turns out, have a good deal of their own healthy fats in them that your body can use to get through those rough patches and, while they not be the most satisfying snack on their own, you might consider topping your salad with them for a little bit of crunch, or pairing them with some berries to make them a little more satisfying.

Probiotics to help boost your gut health.

Probiotics can be found in a number of different ways in health food stores, but they can make digestion and gut health much more optimum. Having a happy gut often means that your dietary success and overall health will improve!

Vegetables that are rich in healthy fats.

Not to sound topical or trendy, but avocados are a great example of a vegetable that is packed with healthy fats. Look for vegetables with fatty acids and a higher fat content and you will find that if you add more of those into your regimen, you will get hungry less often.

Water, water, water, and more water.

No matter what you decide to add to or subtract from your regimen, stay hydrated. This will aid in digestive health and ease, it will keep you from feeling as slumpy or tired, and it will keep you from getting too hungry. Add electrolytes where you need to and don't be shy about bringing a bottle with you when you go from place to place. Stay hydrated!

What to avoid

Grains

While grains may have their health benefits and be full of fiber, you can also get these nutrients elsewhere. The human diet does not require grain consumption. The truth is while grains may have some benefits, they are ridiculously high in both total and net carbohydrates, making them incompatible with the ketogenic diet. A single serving of brown rice contains a shocking forty-two net carbs, which is almost double your net carb intake for an entire day.

Although, some people do try what is known as the targeted ketogenic diet, which is a version of the diet specifically designed for those who complete extended and strenuous workouts. With the targeted ketogenic diet, a person will consume a small serving of a carb-heavy food, such as grains, thirty to forty minutes before working out.

Starchy Vegetables and Legumes

Some vegetables are high in carbohydrates. This includes potatoes, beans, beets, corn, and more. Yes, these vegetables may have nutritional benefits, but you can get these same nutrients in low-carb vegetable alternatives. To put into perspective how high in carbs these options can be, a medium-sized white potato contains forty-three net carbs (more than a serving of brown rice!), a standard sweet potato contains twenty-three net carbs, and a serving of black beans contains twenty-five net carbs.

Sugary Fruits

Most fruits contain a high sugar content, meaning that they are also high in carbohydrates, will spike your blood sugar, and cause an insulin reaction. To avoid this, it is important to avoid most fruits. The exception is that you can enjoy berries, lemons, and limes in moderation. Some people will also enjoy a small serving of melon as a treat from time to time, but watch your portion size as it can add up quickly!

Milk and Low-Fat Dairy Products

As you can enjoy dairy products such as cheese on the ketogenic diet, you may consider trying milk. Sadly, milk is much higher in carbohydrates than cheese, with a glass of two-percent milk containing twelve carbs, half of your daily total. Instead, choose low-carb and dairy-free milk alternatives such as almond, coconut, and soy milk.

You may consider using low-fat cheeses instead of full fat to reduce the saturated fats you are consuming. But, if you are looking to reduce your saturated fat intake, choose lighter cuts of meat rather than low-fat dairy products. The reason for this is because when the cheese is made with low-fat dairy, it naturally has a higher carbohydrate content, which will cut into your daily net carb total.

Cashews, Pistachios, and Chestnuts

While you can enjoy nuts and seeds in moderation, keep in mind that nuts contain a moderate level of carbohydrates, and therefore should be eaten in moderation. However, some nuts are high in carbs and thus are not fed on the ketogenic diet, including cashews, pistachios, and chestnuts.

If you want to enjoy nuts, instead of these options, you can fully enjoy almonds, pecans, walnuts, macadamia nuts, and other options.

Most Natural Sweeteners

While you can certainly enjoy sugar-free natural sweeteners such as stevia, monk fruit, and sugar alcohols, you should avoid natural sweeteners that contain sugar. Suffice to say the sugar content makes these sweeteners naturally high in carbs. But, not only that, they will also spike your blood sugar and insulin. This means you should avoid things such as honey, agave, maple, coconut palm sugar, and dates.

Alcohol

Alcohol is not generally enjoyed on the ketogenic diet, as your body will be unable to burn off calories while your liver attempts to process alcohol. Many people also find that when they are in a state of ketosis, they get drunk more quickly and experience more severe hangovers. Not only that, but alcohol adds unnecessary calories and carbohydrates to your diet.

The worst offenders to choose would be margaritas, piña coladas, sangrias, Bloody Mary, whiskey sours, cosmopolitans, and regular beers.

But, if you do choose to drink alcohol regardless of drink in moderation and choose low-carb versions such as rum, vodka, tequila, whiskey, and gin. The next-best options would be dry wines and light beers.

Chapter 5:Hormonal Health of Women

One of the most dangerous things that women do while they are trying to lose weight is that they ignore the importance of their hormonal health. One of the most significant differences between men and women is the way their bodies treat food. The body of a man doesn't attach too much significance to food. For men, food is just a way to survive. This is in stark contrast to the way the body of a woman treats food. For women, food means much more than simple survival; it is connected to their hormonal balance.

Since the time a girl hits puberty to the time she reaches menopause, her body is physically always in a readiness mode to bear a child. Bearing a child is a big responsibility. A child in the womb is a big drain on the energy sources in a woman's body. Once a woman conceives a child, her body tries its best to provide nutrition to the child. This was always not possible through conventional mediums in the past. In the past, women sometimes got food and most of the time didn't. This can make the survival of the child in the womb difficult. To solve this problem, nature has devised the plan of energy store inside the body to help the child survive. This is the reason women have a comparatively higher body fat ratio than men, and they are also more likely to gain fat rapidly. It is not a weakness they have, but a brilliant plan devised by nature for the survival of the coming generations.

Food and Female Hormones Are Connected

The hormones in the body are chemical messengers that help in passing on vital information to the brain. Hormones regulate several crucial functions. If you look closely, the life of a woman is completely dominated by these hormones.

Thyroid and pituitary are two very important glands that secrete most of the hormones. They also regulate the behavior of a woman. These glands are also present in men but don't have that profound impact on them simply because they are not going to bear a child.

Women feel a very strong connection with food and that's why emotional eating, impulsive eating, celebration eating, and all other forms of eating have such strong meanings for women. For women, food is a part of emotional security as it also helps in the regulation and balancing of certain hormones.

Impact of Calorie-Restrictive Diets of Hormonal Balance

Calorie-restrictive diets can harm the hormonal balance in women. It can fill them with a sense of insecurity, void, and unhappiness. Scientific experiments on mice have shown that prolonged calorie-restriction can also lead to the shrinking of female reproductive organs, and they may also lose their ability to reproduce effectively.

Strict diets can also cause irregular periods, and they may also face problems in conception. Women on calorie-restrictive diets can also experience strong and sudden mood swings and they may also become more temperamental. Anger, frustration, irritation, hopelessness, temptation, and cravings are some of the strong feelings experienced by women when they are on calorie-restrictive diets.

It is very important to understand that hormonal balance is very important. Without the hormonal balance, the overall health of a woman will always remain compromised. This is the problem most women keep facing all their lives.

In the pursuit of weight loss and a slender body, women compromise on their hormonal health and end up paying in the form of problems like PCOS, thyroid, metabolic disorders, and other reproductive issues.

Intermittent Fasting- A Reliable Way to Lose Weight Without Compromising Hormonal Health

Intermittent fasting is a safe way to lose weight as it doesn't force you to compromise with your hormonal health. Intermittent fasting doesn't make you starve for food or limit your calorie intake specifically.

It is a process that allows you to eat reasonably. There are no calorie-restrictions. You can eat whatever you feel like as long as you maintain adequate control over quantity.

This eliminates cravings, temptations, and obsessiveness regarding certain food items, and hence your hormones remain in control.

Intermittent fasting is not about what to eat but when to eat. The most important thing in intermittent fasting is to observe abstinence from food for a certain number of hours every day. This period can be easily timed to be your sleep time, and hence severe hunger pangs, and cravings can easily be avoided.

Chapter 6:Exercising on IF for Women over 50

Many people will ask if it is safe to combine fasting with exercise. I am here to say it is. However, some factors need to be considered before combining the two. First, the type of fasting regimen should be considered alongside the physical, mental, and psychological health of the individual. Women with existing medical conditions should not combine fasting with exercises before being advised by a medical expert. So, while it is safe to practice intermittent fasting and include exercise if you are an already active person, doing so is not suitable for everyone.

First of all, your metabolism can be negatively impacted if you exercise and fast for long periods. For example, if you exercise daily while fasting for more than a month, your metabolic rate can begin to slow down. So, while it may sound like a quick way to reap the benefits of your limited calorie intake, moderation is crucial.

Combining the two can trigger a higher rate of breaking down glycogen and body fat. This means that you burn fat at an accelerated rate. Also, when you combine these two, your growth hormones are boosted. This results in improved bone density. Your muscles are also positively impacted when you exercise. Your muscles will become more resilient to stress and age slower. This is also a quick way to trigger autophagy keeping brain cells and tissues strong, making you feel, and look younger.

Cardiovascular exercise is great for the heart and lungs. It improves oxygen delivery to specific parts of your body, reduces stress, improves sleep, burns fat, and improves sex drive. Among the more common cardio exercises are brisk walking running, , and swimming. In the gym, machines such as the elliptical, treadmill, and Stairmaster are used to help with cardio. Some people are satisfied and feel like they've done enough after 20 minutes on the treadmill, but if you want to continue to be strong and independent as you grow older, you need to consider adding strength training to your workout. After 50, strength training for a woman is no longer about six-pack abs, building biceps, or vanity muscles. Instead, it has switched to maintaining a body that is healthy, strong, and is less prone to injury and illness.

Strength Training Exercises for Women Over 50

These ten strength training exercises you can do right in the comfort of your home. All you need is a mat, a chair, and some hand weights of about 3 – 8 pounds. As you get stronger, you can increase the weight. Take a minute to rest before switching between each routine. Ensure that you move slowly through the exercises, breathe properly, and focus on maintaining the right form. If you start to feel lightheaded or dizzy during your routines, especially if you are performing the exercise during your fasting window, discontinue immediately.

Squat to Chair

This exercise is great for improving your bone health. A lot of age-related bone fractures and falls in women involve the pelvis, so this exercise will target and strengthen your pelvic bone and the surrounding muscles.

To perform this:

1.   Stand fully upright in front of a chair as if you are ready to sit and spread your feet shoulder-width apart.

2.   Extend your arms in front of you and keep them that way all through the movement.

3.   Bend your knees and slowly lower your hips as if you want to sit on the chair, but don't sit. When your butt touches the chair slightly, press into your heels to get back your initial standing position. Repeat that for about 10 to 15 times.

Forearm Plank

This exercise targets your core and shoulders.

Here's how to do it:

1.   Get into a push-up position, but with your arms bent at the elbows such that your forearm is supporting your weight.

2.   Keep your body off the mat or floor and keep your back straight at all times. Don't raise or drop your hips. This will engage your core. Hold the position for 30 seconds and then drop to your knees. Repeat ten times.

Modified Push-ups

This routine targets your arms, shoulders, and core.

How's how to do it:

1.   Kneel on your mat. Place your hands on the mat below your shoulders and let your knees be behind your hips so that your back is stretched at an angle.

2.   Tuck your toes under and tighten your abdominal muscles. Gradually bend your elbows as you lower your chest toward the floor.

3.   Push back on your arms to press your chest back to your previous position. Repeat for as many times as is comfortable.

Bird Dog

When done correctly, this exercise can strengthen the muscles of your posterior chain as it targets your back and core. It may seem easy at first but can be a bit tricky.

To do this correctly:

1.   Go on all fours on your mat.

2.   Tighten your abdominal muscles and shift your weight to your right knee and left hand. Slowly extend your right hand in front of you and your left leg behind you. Ensure that both your hands and legs are extended as far as possible and stay in that position for about 5 seconds. Return to your starting position. This is one repetition. Switch to your left knee and right hand and repeat the movement. Alternate between both sides for 20 repetitions.

Shoulder Overhead Press

This targets your biceps, shoulders, and back.

To perform this move:

1.   With dumbbells in both hands, stand and spread your feet shoulder-width apart.

2.   Bring the dumbbells up to the sides of your head and tighten your abdominal muscles.

3.   Slowly press the dumbbells up until your arms are straight above your head. Slowly return to the first position. Repeat 10 times. You can also do this exercise while sitting.

Chest Fly
This targets your chest, back, core, and glutes.
To do this:
1.   Lie with your back flat on your mat, your knees at an angle close to 90 degrees, and your feet firmly planted on the floor or mat.
2.   Hold dumbbells in both hands over your chest. Keep your palms facing each other and gently open your hands away from your chest. Let your upper arms touch the floor without releasing the tension in them.
3.   Contract your chest muscles and slowly return the dumbbells to the initial position. Repeat for about ten times.

Standing Calf Raise
This exercise improves the mobility of your lower legs and feet and also improves your stability.
Here's how to perform it.
1.   Hold a dumbbell in your left hand and place your right hand on something sturdy to give you balance.
2.   When you are sure of your balance, lift your left foot off the floor with the dumbbell hanging at your side. Stand erect and move your weight such that you are almost standing on your toes.
3.   Slowly return to the starting position. Do this 15 times before switching to the other leg and doing the same thing all over again.

Single-Leg Hamstring Bridge
This move targets your glutes, quads, and hamstrings.
To do this:
1.   Lie flat on your back. Place your feet flat on mat or the floor and spread your bent knees apart.
2.   Place your arms flat by your side and lift one leg straight.
3.   Contract your glutes as you lift your hips into a bridge position with your arms still in position. Hold for about 2 to 3 seconds and drop your hips to the mat. Repeat about ten times before switching your leg. Do the same again.

Bent-Over Row
This targets your back muscles and spine.
To do this:
1.   Hold dumbbells in both hands and stand behind a sturdy object (for example, a chair). Bend forward and rest your head on the chosen object. Relax your neck and slightly bend your knees. With both palms facing each other pull the dumbbells to touch your ribs. Hold the position for about 2 to 5 seconds and slowly return to the starting position. Repeat 10 to 15 times.

Basic Ab
A distended belly is a common occurrence in older women. This exercise can strengthen and tighten the abdominal muscles bringing them inward toward your spine.
To perform this:
1.   Lie on your back with your feet firmly planted on the floor and your knees bent. Relax your upper body and rest your hands on your thighs.

2.   As you exhale, lift yourself upward off the mat or floor. Stop the upward movement when your hands are resting on your knees. Hold the position for about 2 to 5 seconds and then slowly return to the starting position. Repeat for about 20 to 3o times.

Including exercises in your daily routine

You do not have to hit the gym or plan a time dedicated to working out. You can make exercise part of your daily routine so that you are always getting the proper amount of body movement, whether or not it is time for exercise.

Tips on how to include exercises into your daily routine.

•   Take the stairs (within reason) instead of using the elevator. You don't want to go up a ten-story building using the stairs! If you have a long way to go up or down, take the stairs a couple of flights and then complete your trip with the elevator.

•   When you talk with your family members at home, don't shout from the top floor and bottom floor. Go up or climb down and talk with them.

•   Find a sporting activity that you thoroughly enjoy and do it as often as is convenient. When you're doing something you enjoy, you'll hardly think of it as exercise, and you're likely to stay committed.

•   If you are at work, instead of sending emails or text messages to coworkers, walk up to them and talk to them face to face.

•   If possible, convert your one-on-one meetings to a walking meeting. Hold the meeting while taking a stroll outside.

•   Stop a block or two from your destination and walk the rest of the way. Make walking your preferred mode of transportation.

•   Take your dog for walks daily. If you don't have a dog, adopt one. It might seem that you are merely walking your dog, but you are exercising your muscles.

•   Take brisk walks as often as possible. Remember to put on comfortable shoes when walking briskly. You can bring your walking shoes with you to make it easy for you to change into them.

Staying Safe While Combining Intermittent Fasting and Exercise

Exercising in your fasting window can help you quickly achieve some of the advanced benefits of intermittent fasting. Nevertheless, it is crucial to follow a few general guidelines to keep you safe during the practice.

There are no iron-cast rules about when to exercise even on fasting days. Observe what works well for you whether exercising before eating (during the fasting window) or eating before working out (during the eating window). Many women find that exercising on an empty stomach suits their body and leaves them feeling energized for the rest of the day. If this is your, set aside time in the morning before your first meal of the day. Some other women find that although they prefer working out on an empty stomach, they feel depleted right after the exercise. In that case, shift your exercise to about 20 to 30 minutes before your first meal of the day. Your body would have rested a bit after your exercise before you break your fast.

If you prefer working out after you break your fast, that is perfectly fine. Eating shortly before your exercise doesn't render your exercises ineffective. Remember that all of our bodies work in different ways. Keep in mind that the goal of working out is to maintain proper body health long into your golden years. You don't need to impress anyone with great abs or biceps, instead impress yourself with how much power you have. Stay committed to your routines, but don't overdo it. If you start feeling weak, that is your cue to take a break.

If you are fasting for longer periods (24 hours or more), you will need to conserve your energy. Consider doing exercises that will not exert too much stress. Take a walk, do some yoga, or any other type of low-intensity exercise.

We could all use someone on our shoulder reminding us to drink more water. And going without food reduces your body's water content even more. Add in higher levels of exertion and you'll be depleting your water reserves very quickly. So here is your reminder to always drink adequate amounts of water before, during, and after your workout sessions.

Chapter 7: Precautions to Take while on IF

Find a Worthy Goal

First things first: find a goal that is worth pursuing, or else you will drop the idea at the first sign of resistance. If you don't have a goal that represents a strong ideal, it won't be long before you start telling yourself, "I think I've passed the stage of such childishness." And yes, many women start a new lifestyle change for reasons that they can't keep up when things get tough. For example, the desire to look like models on TV, or social media makes losing weight feel socially acceptable, and ok to keep up with trends that can be harmful. These reasons are not enough to keep anyone committed to a full lifestyle change and few wonders why so many people with goals are quick to jump from one lifestyle to another.

Don't go into fasting intermittently because it is the thing to do at the moment. Instead, look for inspiring goals such as:

- Staying fit, young, and healthy.
- Improving your cognitive or brain functions.
- Improving your overall vitality and increase energy levels.
- Balancing hormones, especially during menopausal or post-menopausal stages of life.
- Improving your overall health, thereby increasing longevity.

Do any of these sounds good to you? Surely at this stage of your life, you are aware of the inherent risks of doing something merely because others are doing it too. That type of motivation will fail you.

Check Your Hormones

A woman's hormones can be easily thrown out of whack by the slightest change in her already established pattern of behavior. Whether it is a physical change such as altering you're eating pattern or an emotional change such as being irritated or sad, it can bring about hormonal imbalance in a woman even if it is temporary.

But for the perimenopausal and menopausal women, hormones can go haywire for reasons even they can't define. She could be feeling really great all week, and without anything changing she could suddenly become fatigued, depressed, and not in the right frame of mind. These changes happen due to the unpredictability of this phase of a woman's life. Because this can happen for no apparent reason, it is best to check your hormonal levels before putting your body through a major lifestyle change. If you've ever had issues with thyroid, cortisol, or adrenal fatigue, ensure that you have these checks before you begin.

This could be a surprise to some women, but your ovaries produce testosterone too. So, as you grow older and begin to experience a decline in your estrogen and progesterone levels, your testosterone levels are also taking a nosedive. Your libido can be affected by low levels of testosterone and make you feel exhausted and bummed-out for no reason at all. So, while you are checking your other hormones, don't forget to do a testosterone test. The thyroid and testosterone hormones also help in weight regulation. So, if you intend to shed some weight using intermittent fasting, these tests are very necessary.

Start Slow

To go from having five or six meals daily to eating only once a day can lead to very dire consequences. Apart from being harmful to your health, massive abrupt changes are hardly sustainable. After confirming that intermittent fasting is suitable for your health, the next thing to do is planning how to ease into the habit. Take another look at the example of how to ease into fasting in Chapter 2 and consider following the example or coming up with something similar that works for you. In other words, before you fully implement any intermittent fasting regimen, it is a good practice to first test the waters, so to speak, with a less strict form of fasting. By doing this, it will help your body acclimate to the changes before going into the proper regimen.

Don't Fuss Over What You Can Eat

One common mistake people make when fasting is obsessing over the fasting hours and what to eat when they are finally allowed. You don't have to worry about if you are fasting as long as someone else, the important thing is what's comfortable for you. Of course, if your fasting window is too small, you are not likely to see any result. Also, don't get too tied up in every little detail of intermittent fasting. For example, you don't have to become too worried because you missed a day. Remember that fasting intermittently should be a lifestyle change if you want to continue to reap the benefits. And for a lifestyle change to be sustainable, you must be able to adapt and use it in a way that even if you face challenges, you will work your way around it somehow. Missing a day or cutting your fast short for reasons beyond your control shouldn't get you worked up and worrying about whether you can do the entire plan. Don't give up.

Again, some people focus too much on what they can eat or not eat. For example, "Can I add just a little butter or cream?" "Would it hurt to eat this type of food during the fasting window?" If your focus is on what you can have or eat while you are fasting, you are giving your attention to the wrong things and putting your mind in an unhelpful state. Give your mind the right focus by concentrating on doing a good, clean, fast, and try to consume only water, tea, or coffee during the window.

Watch Electrolytes

Your body electrolytes are compounds and elements that occur naturally in body fluids, blood, and urine. They can also be ingested through drinks, foods, and supplements. Some of them include magnesium, calcium, potassium, chloride, phosphate, and sodium. Their functions include fluid balance, regulation of the heart and neurological function, acid-base balance, oxygen delivery, and many other functions.

It is important to keep these electrolytes in a state of balance. But many people who practice fasting tend to neglect this and run into problems. Here is a common notion: "Don't let anything into your stomach until the end of your fast" Even those just starting to fast know it doesn't work that way, and they tend to forget or fully stay away from liquids during their fasting window.

When you lose too much water from your body through sweating, vomiting, and diarrhea, or you don't have enough water in your body because you don't drink enough liquids, you increase the risk of electrolyte disorders. It is not okay to drink tea or black coffee throughout the morning period of your fast window. You will wear down if you do not drink enough water. The longer you fast without water, the higher your chances of flushing out electrolytes and running into trouble. You can end up raising your blood pressure, develop muscle twitching and spasms, fatigue, fast heart rate or irregular heartbeat, and many other health problems.

In contrast, drinking too much water can also tip the water-electrolyte balance. What you want to do is to drink adequate amounts of water and not excess water, whether you are fasting or not.

Give the Calorie Restriction a Rest

Remember that intermittent fasting is different from dieting. Your focus should be on eating healthily during your eating window or eating days instead of focusing on calorie restriction. Even if you are fasting for weight loss, don't obsess over calories. Following a fasting regimen is enough to take care of the calories you consume. It is absolutely unnecessary to engage in a practice that can hurt your metabolism. Combining intermittent fasting with eating too little food in your eating window because you are worried about your calorie intake can cause problems for your metabolism.

One of the major reasons that people push themselves into restricting calories while fasting is their concern for rapid weight loss. You need to be wary of any process that brings about drastic physical changes to your body in very short amounts of time. While it is okay to desire quick results, your health and safety are more important. When you obsess or worry that you are not losing weight as quickly as you want, you are not helping matters. Instead, you are increasing your stress level, and that is counterproductive. You are already taking practical steps toward losing weight by intermittent fasting, why would you want to undo your hard work by unnecessary worrying?

Simply focus on following a sustainable intermittent fasting regimen and let go of the need to restrict your calorie intake. Intermittent fasting will give your body the right number of calories it needs if you do it properly.

The First Meal of the Eating Window Is Key

Breaking your fast is a crucial part of the process because if you don't get it right, it could quickly develop into unhealthy eating patterns. When you break your fast, it is important to have healthy foods around to prevent grabbing unhealthy feel good snacks. Make sure what you are eating in your window is not a high-sugar or high-carb meal. I recommend that you consider breaking your fast with something that is highly nutrient-dense such as a green smoothie, protein shake, or healthy salad.

As much as possible, avoid breaking your fast with foods from a fast-food restaurant. Eating junk foods after your fast is a quick way to ruin all the hard work you've put in during your fasting window. If, for any reason, you can't prepare your meal, ensure that you order very specific foods that will complement your effort and not destroy what you've built.

Break Your Fast Gently

It is okay to feel very hungry after going for a long time without food, even if you were drinking water all through the fasting window. This is particularly true for people who are just starting with fasting. But don't let the intensity of your hunger

31

push you to eat. You don't want to force food hurriedly into your stomach after going long without food, or you might hurt yourself and experience stomach distress. Take it slow when you break your fast. Eat light meals in small portions first when you break your fast. Wait for a couple of minutes for your stomach to get used to the presence of food again before continuing with a normal-sized meal. The waiting period will douse any hunger pangs and remove the urge to rush your meal. For example, break your fast with a small serving of salad and wait for about 15 minutes. Drink some water and then after about five more minutes, you can eat a normal-sized meal.

Nutrition is Important

Although intermittent fasting is not dieting and so, does not specify which foods to eat, limit, and completely avoid, it makes sense to eat healthily. This means focusing on eating a balanced diet, such as:

- Whole grains
- Fruits and vegetables (canned in water, fresh, or frozen).
- Lean sources of protein (lentils, beans, eggs, poultry, tofu, and so on).
- Healthy fats (nuts, seeds, coconuts, avocados, olive oil, olive, and fatty fish).

It simply doesn't make any sense to go for 16 hours (or more) without food and then spend the rest of the day eating junk. Even if you follow the 5:2 diet and limit your calorie intake to only 500 calories per day for two days, it is totally illogical to follow it with five days of eating highly processed foods and low-quality meals. Combining intermittent fasting with unbalanced diets will lead to nutritional deficiencies and defeat the goal of fasting in the first place. Realize that intermittent fasting is not a magic wand that makes all poor eating habits vanish in a poof! For the practice to work, you must be deliberate about the types of food you eat.

Find a Regimen That Works for You

Don't follow a fasting diet because it seems to suit someone else. Instead, go for something that fits into your schedule. If you feel caged or boxed in by a particular fasting plan, it is a clear indication that it is not a suitable plan for you. Thankfully, you have the freedom to design something that works for you, even if you are following a specific regimen. The regimens are not carved in stone! They are flexible, and you can adjust them to suit you as long as you follow each regimen's basic principles. For example, if you decide to follow the 16:8 fasting regimen, your 8-hour eating window must not strictly be between noon and 8 pm. You have the option of tailoring the eating window to something that gives you room to handle other aspects of your life, such as work, hobbies, family, and so on. You might decide to make your 8-hour eating window from 9 am to 5 pm, or from 1 pm to 9 pm. Whatever you choose to do is totally up to you. After all, it is your life, and you have the freedom to choose what you want. Books, the internet, and even loved ones can only suggest and offer recommendations. Ultimately, the final decision rests with you. Since your goal is not to please someone else or seek external approval, you should make your choice based on what is most convenient for you. You are seeking results, not accolades. Therefore, don't follow something unrealistic for you or too restrictive. Even if you endure the most stringent type of fast and get admiration and commendation from others, have you considered what that fasting regimen is doing to your overall health? The female body is delicately designed, and putting it through unnecessary stress is unsafe if you are merely enduring discomfort to boost your ego.

Be Patient

Whatever propaganda you may have heard about fast results, the reality is that nothing is typical because we all have unique processes regardless of our physical appearance. Be patient even if others who began fasting at the same time are already seeing results and you have nothing to show for your efforts so far. It can be frustrating and discouraging but give your body time to adjust. As long as you don't have any medical reason to stop, don't give up just yet. Continue the practice for at least a month.

Realize that changes take time. There is no magic about the process of losing weight, improved vitality, or any other health benefits of intermittent fasting. Don't be in a hurry, and don't give people the room to put you under unnecessary pressure. Each person has their own pace, and it has absolutely nothing to do with you. If you continue to focus on other people's results or your seeming lack of results, you are giving your mind reasons to discontinue. Be patient.

Myths about intermittent fasting

Skipping breakfast makes you fat

One progressing fantasy is that morning meal is the most significant feast of the day. Individuals normally accept that skipping breakfast prompts unnecessary yearning, desires, and weight gain. One 16-week study in 283 grown-ups with overweight and heftiness watched no weight distinction between the individuals who had breakfast and the individuals who didn't. Consequently, breakfast doesn't generally influence your weight, despite the fact that there might be some individual changeability. A few examinations even recommend that individuals who get thinner over the long haul will in general have breakfast. Also, kids and young people who have breakfast will, in general, perform better at school. Thusly, it's imperative to focus on your specific needs. Breakfast is gainful for certain individuals, while others can skip it with no negative outcomes.

Eating much of the time supports your digestion

Numerous individuals accept that eating more dinners builds your metabolic rate, making your body consume more calories overall. Your body surely consumes a few calories processing suppers. This is named the thermal impact of nourishment. By and large, TEF utilizes around 10% of your complete calorie consumption. Nonetheless, what is important is the absolute number of calories you expend not what number of suppers you eat. Eating six 500-calorie dinners has a similar impact as eating three 1,000-calorie suppers. Given a normal TEF of 10%, you'll consume 300 calories in the two cases.

Various investigations exhibit that expanding or diminishing dinner recurrence doesn't influence complete calories consumed.

Eating much of the time diminishes hunger

A few people accept that occasional eating forestalls yearnings and exorbitant appetite. However, the proof is blended. Albeit a few investigations propose that eating increasingly visit dinners prompts decreased yearning, different examinations have discovered no impact or even expanded appetite levels.

One investigation that thought about eating three or six high-protein meals every day found that eating three dinners decreased yearning all the more successfully. All things considered; reactions may rely upon the person. In the event that regular eating lessens your yearnings, it's most likely a smart thought. All things considered, there's no proof that eating or eating more often reduces hunger for everybody.

Visit dinners can assist you with shedding pounds

Since eating all the more as often as possible doesn't support your digestion, it moreover doesn't have any impact on weight reduction. In reality, an examination in 16 grown-ups with stoutness thought about the impacts of eating 3 and 6 meals per day and found no distinction in weight, fat misfortune, or craving.

A few people guarantee that eating frequently makes it harder for them to hold fast to a healthy diet. Nevertheless, on the off chance that you find that eating all the more frequently makes it simpler for you to eat less calories and less lousy nourishment, don't hesitate to stay with it.

Irregular fasting causes you to lose muscle

A few people accept that when you quick, your body begins consuming muscle for fuel. In spite of the fact that this occurs with eating less junk food when all is said in done, no proof recommends that it happens more with irregular fasting than different strategies. Then again, considers demonstrate that irregular fasting is better for keeping up bulk. Strikingly, irregular fasting is well known among many bodybuilders, who find that it keeps up muscle close by a low muscle to fat ratio.

Irregular fasting is awful for your wellbeing

While you may have heard bits of gossip that irregular fasting hurts your wellbeing, examines uncover that it has several impressive medical advantages. For instance, it changes your quality articulation identified with life span and resistance and has been appeared to draw out life expectancy in creatures.

It additionally has significant advantages for metabolic wellbeing, for example, improved insulin sensitivity and diminished oxidative pressure, irritation, and coronary illness chance. It might likewise support cerebrum wellbeing by raising degrees of mind inferred neurotrophic factor (BDNF), a hormone that may secure against melancholy and different other states of mind.

Various fantasies get propagated about intermittent fasting and feast recurrence. Be that as it may, a large number of these bits of gossip are not valid. For instance, eating littler, increasingly visit dinners doesn't support your digestion or assist you with shedding pounds. In addition, discontinuous fasting is a long way from undesirable and may offer various advantages. It's essential to counsel sources or do a little research before forming a hasty opinion about your metabolism and generally speaking wellbeing.

Chapter 8:Mistakes to Avoid

Starting intermittent fasting quickly

Many beginners make the mistake of starting intermittent fasting way too fast, and when they begin to quickly, it becomes unsustainable for them to continue with intermittent fasting. If you have started anything immediately, you might have noticed that it became tough for you to follow, which led to you not continuing. Same goes for intermittent fasting, and you need to make sure you take the right steps before you jump into following intermittent fasting. With that being said, let's talk about many ways beginner intermittent fasters tend to start too quickly. The first mistake they make is by picking a fasting protocol, which is way out of their Realm. As we talked about before, you need to ease into intermittent fasting, especially if you're women. You cannot expect to fast for 24 hours when you have never even fasted in your life, so start small. It is always recommended that women begin with 12-hour fast, or if that sounds too intense for you can start to by meal skipping. You have to make sure that, whatever you follow it is done gradually, so you don't quit. Another way people tend to start intermittent fasting too quickly is by not Consulting the doctor. Believe it or not, their chances that you might not be healthy enough to follow intermittent fasting.

That is why it is advised that you consult a doctor before starting fasting; for example, if you have diabetes, you are not advised to begin intermittent fasting. There are many health complications which not allow you to follow intermittent fasting, that is why we always recommend you ask a doctor before you start intermittent fasting or it can be very devastating.

Beginners also tend to extend the fasting window very quickly; if you haven't fasted for more than four weeks comfortably, then it is not recommended to extend the fasting window. We need to take into consideration that for beginners, going from 12 hours to 16 hours can be a drastic difference. That is why you stick with a fasting protocol for an extended period, ideally for four weeks. If you make the jump of increasing hours too soon, you will notice it becomes tough for you to continue with fasting and you might give up.

Choosing the wrong plan for your lifestyle

Most people, when they first start intermittent fasting, tend to pick the crazy strategy for their lifestyle. It is important that you choose the right method for your lifestyle and your goals. Intermittent fasting can be very fitting for most lifestyle. However, some plans are just better suited for some. Which is what we are going to be talking about in this section of the book, picking the right plan for your lifestyle. To simplify this process, we will make up two people and make up a fake lifestyle. Once we have managed to do that, we will figure out which fasting protocol works best for them

Overeating during the eating window or too little

People make the mistake of eating a lot or too little when following intermittent fasting, and the truth is it is straightforward to do either. People who are looking to lose weight will eat less during their eating window, thinking that it will help you lose more body fat. Whereas overeating will not make up for all the fasting, you did throughout the day. Which is why it is imperative that you do none, so in this section, we will teach you how to make sure you aren't doing either when following an intermittent fasting protocol.

The first way to not mess up on overeating would be to make sure that you are counting your macros. This is among the best ways to make sure you stay on track with your eating habits during your fasting windows. When you have calculated your macros and following them accordingly, you will have a lot better chance of not under eating or overeating during your eating window. Another way to make sure that you are not overeating is to eat slowly, and many people tend to get extremely excited when they see food in front of them during their eating window. It is best advised that you don't indulge in them and more than you should.

This is the reason why it is essential that you control your cravings; we have taught you how to do that in the previous chapters. Now, even though fasting allows you to eat whatever you want when you break your fast, it still essential to make sure you eat correctly. You see if you try and eat junk food and try and hit your macros, it would be tough for you not to overeat. Let me explain how that works, as there is something called a high glycemic carb which most of the junk foods. What these high glycemic carbs are responsible for is digesting very quickly in your body, which spikes the insulin very fast.

When you absorb and shuttle the foods to quickly as you would with junk food, you will get hungry very fast, which would make you overeat. Which is why it is best advised that you eat foods which have a lower glycemic index like most healthy meals tend to have. Another thing these healthy foods will help you with would be the fiber, making you feel fuller through the day. Now that we know how not to overeat, let's talk about how to make sure that you aren't under-eating. The first way to make sure that you aren't under-eating would be by counting macros, and this will help you make sure that you are hitting all your calories for the day. Counting macros will ensure you don't under-eat and you don't overeat, it goes hand in hand.

Now, this is the only way to avoid under-eating let's talk about some of the signs you might be experiencing if you under-eat when fasting. The first sign you might notice is that you feel very weak when working out if you follow a workout plan you will see that your strength has gone down which is a tail-tail sign that you are under-eating. Another way to tell that you are under-eating is if you know that you feel less energy throughout the day, rather than feeling more heat. One of the many benefits of intermittent fasting is the fact that you can get a lot more power, but it won't work if you are under-eating. So, by now, you can tell that overeating and under-eating aren't optimal for fasting. Which is why you need to make sure that you stay on track with your macros when fasting, the other tips we gave you work great as well.

But do whatever works for you to ensure that you aren't under eating or overeating, and there are millions of ways to go about it. Find an eating routine which helps you feel full, and allows you to eat just the right amount of calories to where you are getting closer to your goals instead of drifting away from them if your goal is weight loss or muscle gains you need to make sure your calories are the right amount. Don't make this beginners mistake as you will regret it, and now you have the tools to ensure you don't make these mistakes.

Ignoring what for when

One mistake that many people following intermittent fasting make is to ignore what for when. For you to be successful with intermittent fasting, you need to make sure you don't overlook what for when. What do I mean by what for when is simple, ignoring what to do and what not to do when intermittent fasting? We will talk about things to avoid and the things not to avoid when intermittent fasting. More specifically, we will teach you how to listen to your body.

You are ignoring what for when is merely a metaphor, nonetheless an important one. First of all, when intermittent fasting doesn't jump too quickly from fasts to fasts. Most beginners make the mistake of not riding out the protocol for a substantial amount of time before they jump to conclusions. Make sure that you have done at least four weeks of following this protocol as it will show you how your body reacts to this fasting method. The next thing to make sure of would be to understand how your body reacts to certain types of fasting, as it is essential that you know so. Before you jump the guns of upping the fasting difficultly, make sure you know how your body works. You need to remember that your body is more important than your goals, so whatever you do, you need to be aware of what your body is telling you. Don't do anything which makes you feel like you are harming your body, and as always consult with your physician before you start a fast.

Not drinking enough water

Drinking water is crucial when your intermittent fasting, is there a lot of benefits to drinking water. It also helps you care about your appetite. We will talk about the reasons why you should be drinking more water when intermittent fasting, and also show you why you might not be drinking enough water and techniques to allow you to drink more water when fasting. Many people know that water is very beneficial to humans, water help to detox your body clean out your system and also helps you curb appetite. It is crucial that you're drinking more water when fasting. Believe it or not, most of the time you're drinking a lot less water than you required to be drinking. One of the best rules of thumb to follow when you are drinking water is too drink 1 oz per pound of body weight. So, if you weigh 150 lbs., you should be drinking 150 ounces of water, especially when you're intermittent fasting; as water will help you forget about food.

Many people know that when you're fasting, especially in the beginning you tend to crave a lot of food. What water will do is help you curb that appetite, so you don't break you're fast prematurely, another thing water will do detoxify your body. When your fasting you're already detoxing a lot of things, if you add more water to it, it will help you detox your body even further making it a lot healthier environment for you. Water will also increase your brain power and productivity, as you know intermittent fasting has shown to improve mental focus so once you add more water to your daily routine, you will notice more focused throughout the day.

Another thing water helps you with is that it helps you lose body weight. If you started intermittent fasting in the hopes of losing weight, then you need to drink more water. What water does, is it increase your metabolism, which equals more calories burnt throughout the day. Water will also help you clean out your complexion, so if that's what you're looking for the water will help you with that. Intermittent fasting has shown to improve with your digestive system, but once you add a sufficient amount of water to it will boost it further. Many people know that regularity in the essential thing when it comes to a healthy body, why do I help you with consistency, which will equal a better digestive system and overall well-being. Water will also help you boost your immune system, as it enables you to clean out your toxins.

When incorporated with intermittent fasting, drink more water to boost your immune system. When fasting, you might notice headaches, especially in the beginning, if you drink a sufficient amount of water throughout the day, you will not see problems. Headaches is one of the biggest concerns when fasting, many people notice problems, and to avoid that you should start drinking more water. Another matter that you might see when fasting is cramped more specifically muscle cramps. One of the ways to prevent it is to drink more water. Now I can keep going on with the benefits of drinking more water, but you get the idea to drink more water to avoid side effects from fasting that you might see.

One of the ways to ensure that you drink more water is to buy a water bottle with markings on it. First, determine how much water you need through the day and make sure you achieve your goal of drinking a set amount of water. Another way to ensure that you drink more water is to set alarms. What many people do, set alerts on this Smartphone, and when the alarm goes off the drink a glass of water. You can do the same thing to ensure they drink enough water throughout the day, calculate the number of glasses you need to achieve your water intake goal, and then set your timer.

Choose whichever method you want to make sure that you're drinking enough water throughout the day. Not drinking enough water is among the biggest mistakes most people make. Our body is made up of around 70% water, and to ignore that and not drink enough water and hinder your progress. Make sure you're drinking enough water, during your fast and after you break your fast. To ensure that you are optimizing your fasting endeavors and getting closer to your goals.

Don't be greedy in festive windows
The food has its temptation. It seems the most attractive in the world when it has been private for a long time. This would also happen to you. But it is vital not to be greedy in those moments and lose control. It is very important to leave the windows fasting properly. The biggest mistake people make is that they eat a lot after breaking the fast. This can cause several problems, and poor digestion is one of them. On an empty stomach, the intestine stays away from food for prolonged periods and, therefore, can dry up a bit. Filling it with heavy foods can cause problems. The best way to start the day is to start with liquid foods and then switch to semi-solid and solid. You should also consider the amount of food you eat. Our brain takes much longer to understand the signs of leptin that is full. When your brain tells you that you are full, you would have eaten too much. The best way out is to eat slowly, as this would give the brain time to assess satiety levels. You can also stop eating when you think it is 80% full.

All in all, you would have eaten enough. If you want to try this, you can wait a while after feeling 80% full, and you will discover that you are no longer hungry. It occurs when fat cells can communicate properly with the brain that it is no longer necessary to eat.

Do not try to speed up the process.

Slow and steady wins the race. This is an adage that we have all heard, but most of us do not believe it. We want fast results, and for this, we are ready to jump. However, this is not how the body works. Your body travels very slowly. You need time to adapt to any positive or negative change, and the same would happen even in the case of intermittent fasting. If you want to succeed with the process, you must make sure you complete all the steps for a while. You have to give your body time to adapt. There would be habits of decades that should change, and sometimes it can be difficult for your body. If you want your body to react favorably to change, you should not rush the process. Fasting in men and women is completely different. Men have a very resistant system and are not affected by a slightly extended rapid program. However, this is not the case with women. If you try to shake the system a little harder, this can negatively affect your health. Your hormonal system can change, and normalization can take a long time. A woman's body reacts very differently to the signs of stress and, therefore, caution and patience are essential. Start with the simplest process and give your body time to adapt to small breaks. Once you are accustomed to a certain amount of brake, try to stretch it a bit slowly. Do not do anything very fast. Always go step by step, and you will get your goal easily and without unnecessary difficulties.

Perseverance is the key

Impatience is a big problem in people struggling with weight. There is no fault of them since they are subject to strong pressure. Most people trying to lose weight have already faced disappointments with other weight loss measures and, therefore, want to see the results quickly to believe it. They are not ready to wait long for the results. This is a point where problems can occur. Intermittent fasting is not a wonderful process. It is a wonderful process, but it does not work by magic. Try to correct problems that may have reached their current state of development in at least decades. The results would take time to arrive. You will have to work with patience and not lose hope when the results arrive. If you stop smoking in the middle, you cannot know if you are progressing or not. It is not a process that works overnight. A leap of faith will be required, and you will devote your time and energy.

Don't frame unrealistic expectations

We all like to dream big, and that is a good thing. However, we must also remain based on reality. This will help to accept the facts and save many disappointments. Many times, we are so caught up in imaginary expectations that we don't recognize the gifts we receive. If your goal is weight loss, think about the amount of time you are ready to devote, the distances you can travel, and the medical conditions you face. Without considering all these facts, expecting a complete makeover would be absurd. If you have met these expectations, you will not even be able to enjoy the weight loss you are observing. Your expectations would overshadow the results. It is important to stay realistic.

Properly manage your fasting time

It is common for some people to mishandle their time. Many of us do it in our daily lives. However, bad time management can cause serious difficulties. It can make your weight loss journey difficult and painful. You can't keep thinking about food while you fast. This would create problems for you, and your gut would also be confused. The best way to manage your fasting time is to keep busy. The last part of the fasting window should always be programmed to remain locked correctly. The more inactive it is, the more likely it is to think only of food. Performing intense physical activity is one of the best ways to postpone hunger. Hunger in the current era is a highly psychological phenomenon. Our bodies have ample reserves of energy to function without food for months. It is our mind that always attracts us to food. You have to stop it for a few hours. Walking, running, laughing, talking with friends, starting serious discussions are some of the ways we can stop hunger and not be affected. These are among the most common mistakes we make that can ruin the results we get. Intermittent fasting is a very simple and easy way to lose weight. It doesn't take much time and effort. You only have to decide once and take it in your life. Even if you are following some other measure of weight loss, intermittent fasting can adapt to your lifestyle.

Chapter 9:The Recipes
Breakfast

Avocado Egg Bowls
Prep time: 5 minutes
Cook time: 10 minutes
Serves: 3
Ingredients:
- 1 tsp coconut oil
- 2 organics, free-range
- Salt and pepper
- 1 Large & ripe avocado

For Garnishing:
- Chopped walnuts
- Balsamic Pearls
- Fresh thyme

Directions:
1. Slice your avocado in two, then take out the pit and remove enough of the inside so that there is enough space inside to accommodate an entire egg.
2. Cut off a little bit of the bottom of the avocado so that the avocado will sit upright as you place it on a stable surface.
3. Open your eggs and put each of the yolks in a separate bowl or container. Place the egg whites in the same small bowl. Sprinkle some pepper and salt to the whites, according to your personal taste, then mix them well.
4. Melt the coconut oil in a pan that has a lid that fits and put it on med-high.
5. Put in the avocado boats, with the meaty side down on the pan, the skin side up and sauté them for approx. 35 seconds, or when they become darker in color.
6. Turn them over, then add to the spaces inside, almost filling the inside with the whites of the eggs.
7. Then, reduce the temperature and place the lid. Let them sit covered it for approx. 16 to 20 minutes until the whites are just about fully cooked.
8. Gently add one yolk onto each of the avocados and keep cooking them for 4 to 5 mins, just until they get to the point of cook you want them at.
9. Move the avocados to a dish and add toppings to each of them using the walnuts, the balsamic pearls, or/and thyme.

Nutritional Information:
Calories 215
Fat 18g
Carbohydrates 8g
Protein 9g

Buttery Date Pancakes

Prep time: 10 minutes
Cook time: 10 minutes
Serves: 3

Ingredients:

- 1/4 cup almond flour
- 3 eggs, beaten
- 1 teaspoon olive oil
- 6 dates, pitted
- 1 tablespoon almond butter
- 1 teaspoon vanilla extract
- 1/2 teaspoon ground cinnamon

Directions:

1. Stir the eggs in a bowl make them fluffy.
2. Wash the dates and cut them in half.
3. Discard the seeds and mash them finely.
4. Melt the almond butter and add to the eggs.
5. Add the almond flour, olive oil and cinnamon.
6. Mix well and add the vanilla extract.
7. Mix into a smooth batter.
8. Add the date paste and mix well.
9. In a pan heat the butter over medium heat.
10. Add the batter using a spoon and fry them golden brown from both sides.
11. Repeat with all the batter.
12. Serve with melted butter on top.

Nutritional information:

Calories 281
Fat 20g
Protein 10.5g
Carbohydrates 4.5g

Low Carb Pancake Crepes

Prep time: 10 minutes
Cook time: 10 minutes
Serves: 2

Ingredients

- 3 ounces cream cheese
- 1 tsp ground cinnamon
- 1 tbsp honey
- 1 tsp ground cardamom
- 1 tsp butter
- 2 egg, beaten

Directions:

1. In a bowl, whisk the eggs finely.
2. Beat the cream cheese in a different bowl until it becomes soft.
3. Add the egg mixture to the softened cream cheese and mix well until there are no lumps left.
4. Add cinnamon, cardamom, and honey to it. Mix well. The batter would be runnier than of pancake batter.
5. In a pan add the butter and heat over medium heat.
6. Add the batter using a scooper, that way all the size of the crepes would be the same.
7. Fry them golden brown on both sides.
8. Repeat the process with the rest of the batter.
9. Drizzle some honey on top and enjoy.

Nutritional information:

Calories 241
Fats 21.8 g
Carbohydrates 2.4g
Proteins 9.6 g

Chia Seed Banana Blueberry Delight

Prep time: 30 minutes

Serves: 2

Ingredients

- 1 cup yogurt
- ½ cup blueberries
- 1/2 tsp Salt
- 1/2 tsp Cinnamon
- 1 banana
- 1 tsp Vanilla Extract
- 1/4 cup Chia Seeds

Directions:

1. Discard the skin of the banana.
2. Cut into semi thick circles.
3. You can mash them or keep them as whole if you like to bite into your fruits.
4. Clean the blueberries properly and rinse well.
5. Soak the chia seeds in water for 30 minutes or longer.
6. Drain the chia seeds and transfer into a bowl.
7. Add the yogurt and mix well.
8. Add the salt, cinnamon and vanilla and mix again.
9. Now fold in the bananas and blueberries gently.
10. If you want add dried fruit or nuts, add it and then serve immediately.
11. This is best served cold.

Nutritional Information:

Calories 260

Fats 26.6g

Carbohydrates 17.4g

Protein 4.1g

Egg Omelet

Prep time: 10 minutes
Cook time: 10 minutes
Serves: 2

Ingredients

- 1 cup cherry tomatoes
- 2 sausage, cooked
- 1 cup spinach
- ½ tsp oregano
- Salt to taste
- Pepper to taste
- 2 eggs
- 2 tbsp heavy cream
- 2 tbsp butter, melted

Directions:

1. Finely chop the cherry tomatoes.
2. Cut off the stem of the spinach. Chop them finely.
3. Crumble the sausage using hands.
4. Mix the eggs with heavy cream in a bowl and add to the skillet.
5. Top the egg with cherry tomatoes, spinach, oregano and sausage.
6. Season using pepper and salt
7. Fold the omelet carefully.
8. Serve with more oregano on top.

Nutritional Information:

Calories 289
Fats 53.9g
Carbohydrates 7.9g
Protein 19.3g

Savory Breakfast Muffins

Prep time: 10 minutes
Cook time: 35 minutes
Serves: 6

Ingredients

- 8 eggs
- 1 cup shredded cheese
- Salt and pepper to taste
- ½ tsp baking powder
- ¼ cup diced onion
- 2/3 cup coconut flour
- 1 ½ cup spinach
- ¼ cup full fat coconut milk
- 1 tbsp basil, chopped
- ½ cup cooked chicken, diced finely

Directions:

1. Preheat the oven to 375-degree F.
2. Use butter or oil to grease your muffin tray or you can use muffin paper liners.
3. In a large mixing bowl, whisk the eggs.
4. Add in the coconut milk and mix again.
5. Gradually shift in the coconut flour with baking powder salt.
6. Add in the cooked chicken, onion, spinach, basil and combine well.
7. Add the cheese and mix again.
8. Pour the mixture onto your muffin liners.
9. Bake for about 25 minutes.
10. Serve in room temperature.

Nutritional Information:

Calories 388
Fat 25.8g
Carbohydrate 8.6g
Proteins 25.3g

Green Pineapple

Prep time: 5 minutes
Cook time: 0 minutes
Serves: 3

Ingredients:

- 1/2 of a pineapple
- 1 broccoli, diced
- 1 cup water
- 1 long cucumber, diced
- A dash of salt
- 1 kiwi, diced

Directions

1. Add kiwi, cucumber, pineapple, broccoli and water in a blender.
2. Add the salt and blend until smooth.
3. Serve.

Nutritional Information:

Calories 251
Fats 0.4g
Proteins 0.5g
Carbohydrates 22g

Wholesome Mushroom and Cauliflower Risotto

Prep time: 15 minutes
Cook time: 10 minutes
Serves: 4

Ingredients:

- 1 medium cauliflower head, cut into florets
- 1 pound of shiitake mushrooms, sliced
- 3 medium garlic cloves, peeled and minced
- 2 tablespoons of coconut aminos
- 1 cup of homemade low-sodium chicken stock
- 1 cup of full-fat coconut milk
- 1 tablespoon of coconut oil, melted
- 1 small onion, finely chopped
- 2 tablespoons of almond flour
- ¼ cup of nutritional yeast

Directions:

1. On the Instant Pot, press "Sauté"and add the coconut oil.
2. Once hot, add the garlic, mushrooms and onions. Sauté for 5 minutes or until softened, stirring occasionally.
3. Add the remaining ingredients except for the almond flour. Cover and cook for 2 minutes on high pressure.
4. When done, release the pressure naturally and remove the lid.
5. Sprinkle the almond flour over the risotto and stir to thicken. Serve and enjoy!

Nutritional Information:

Calories 230
Carbohydrates 8g
Protein 7.5g
Fats 18g

Morning Meatloaf

Prep time: 10 minutes
Cook time: 20 minutes
Serves: 6

Ingredients:

- 1 ½ pound of breakfast sausage
- 6 large organic eggs
- 2 tablespoons of unsweetened non-dairy milk
- 1 small onion, finely chopped
- 2 medium garlic cloves, peeled and minced
- 4-ounces of cream cheese, softened and cubed
- 1 cup of shredded cheddar cheese
- 2 tablespoons of scallions, chopped
- 1 cup of water

Directions:

1.   Add all the ingredients apart from water in a large bowl. Stir until well combined.
2.   Form the sausage mixture into a meatloaf and wrap with a sheet of aluminum foil. Ensure that the meatloaf fits inside your Instant Pot. If not, remove parts of the mixture and reserve for future use.
3.   Once you wrap the meatloaf into a packet, add 1 cup of water and a trivet to your Instant Pot. Put the meatloaf on the trivet's top.
4.   Cover and cook for 25 minutes on high pressure. When done, quick release the pressure. Carefully remove the lid.
5.   Unwrap the meatloaf and check if the meatloaf is done. Serve and enjoy!

Nutritional Information:

Calories 592
Carbohydrates 2.5g
Proteins 11g
Fats 49.5g

Keto Oatmeal

Prep time: 10 minutes
Cook time: 5 minutes
Serves: 2

Ingredients:

- 1 cup of unsweetened coconut milk
- 1 tablespoon coconut butter or ghee
- 1 tablespoon whole flax seeds
- 1 tablespoon chia seeds
- 1 tablespoon sunflower seeds
- 1/8 teaspoons fine sea salt
- Blueberries (for garnish)

Directions:

1. Put all the ingredients into the Instant Pot and mix.
2. Cover and cook for 3 minutes on high pressure.
3. When done, quick release the pressure and remove the lid.
4. Transfer to a bowl and top with blueberries. Serve and enjoy!

Nutritional Information:

Calories 353
Fats 37.2g
Carbohydrates 4.1g
Proteins 3.7g

Cinnamon and Pecan Porridge

Prep time: 10 minutes
Cook time: 10 minutes
Serves: 2

Ingredients:

- 1 cup unsweetened coconut milk
- ¼ cup almond butter
- 1 tablespoon coconut oil, melted
- 2 tablespoons whole chia seeds
- 2 tablespoons hemp seeds
- ¼ cup pecans, chopped
- ¼ cups walnuts, chopped
- ¼ cups unsweetened and toasted coconut
- 1 teaspoon cinnamon

Directions:

1. Put all the ingredients to the Instant Pot and mix.
2. Cover and cook for 9 minutes on high pressure.
3. When done, release the pressure naturally and remove the lid. Serve and enjoy!

Nutritional Information:

Calories 580
Carbohydrates 11g
Protein 32g
Fats 51.7g

Awesome Oatmeal

Prep time: 5 minutes
Cook time: 10 minutes
Serves: 4

Ingredients:

- 1 cup unsweetened coconut flakes
- 2 tablespoons butter or coconut oil
- ½ cup hemp seeds
- 2 tablespoons coconut flour
- 1 cup water
- 2/3 cups coconut cream
- ½ tablespoon ground cinnamon
- 1 teaspoon pure vanilla extract
- 1 tablespoon pure pumpkin pureed
- 1 teaspoon finely grated ginger
- A small pinch fine sea salt

Directions:

1. Put all the ingredients to the Instant Pot and give a good stir.
2. Cover and cook for 9 minutes on high pressure. When done, allow for a full natural release. Carefully remove the lid.
3. Stir the oatmeal again and allow to cool. Serve and enjoy!

Nutritional Information:

Calories 375
Carbohydrates 4g
Protein 12g
Fat 33g

Lunch

Zuppa Toscana with Cauliflower

Prep time: 5 minutes
Cook time: 25 minutes
Serves: 4

Ingredients:

- 1-pound ground Italian sausage
- 6 cups homemade low-sodium chicken stock
- 2 cups cauliflower florets - 1 onion, finely chopped
- 1 cup kale, stemmed and roughly chopped
- 1 (14.5-ounce) can of full-fat coconut milk
- ¼ teaspoon sea salt
- ¼ teaspoon freshly cracked black pepper

Directions:

1. On the Instant Pot, press "Sauté"and add the ground Italian sausage. Cook until brown, stirring occasionally and breaking up the meat with a wooden spoon.
2. Add the remaining ingredients except for the kale and coconut milk and stir until well combined.
3. Cover and cook for 10 minutes on high pressure. When done, release the pressure naturally and remove the lid. Stir in the kale and coconut milk. Cover and sit for 5 minutes or until the kale has wilted. Serve and enjoy!

Nutritional Information:

Calories 653
Carbohydrates 8g
Protein 26g
Fat 4g

Pork Carnitas

Prep time: 20 minutes
Cook time: 1 hour
Serves: 4

Ingredients:

- 6 medium garlic cloves, minced
- 2 teaspoons ground cumin
- 1 teaspoon smoked paprika
- 3 chipotle peppers in adobo sauce, minced
- 1 teaspoon dried oregano
- 2 bay leaves
- 1 cup homemade low-sodium chicken broth
- Fine sea salt and freshly cracked black pepper
- 2 tablespoons of olive oil
- 2 ½ pounds boneless pork shoulder, cut into 4 large pieces

Directions:

1. Season the pork shoulder with sea salt, black pepper, ground cumin, dried oregano, and smoked paprika.
2. On the Instant Pot, press "Sauté" and add the olive oil.
3. Once hot, add the pork pieces and sear for 4 minutes per side or until brown.
4. Add the remaining ingredients inside your Instant Pot. Cover and cook for 80 minutes on high pressure. When done, quick release the pressure and remove the lid.
5. Carefully shred the pork using two forks and continue to stir until well coated with the liquid.
6. Remove the bay leave and adjust the seasoning if necessary. Serve and enjoy!

Nutritional Information:

Calories 170
Carbohydrates 2g
Protein 4g
Fat 8g

Garlic Butter Beef Steak

Prep time: 5 minutes
Cook time: 15 minutes
Serves: 2

Ingredients:

- 1-pound beef sirloin steaks
- ½ cup red wine
- 4 tablespoons unsalted butter
- 2 tablespoons fresh parsley, finely chopped
- 4 medium garlic cloves, peeled and minced
- Fine sea salt and freshly cracked black pepper

Directions:

1. Season the beef steaks with sea salt and freshly cracked black pepper.
2. On the Instant Pot, press "Sauté" and add the butter. Once melted, add the beef steaks and sear for 2 minutes per side or until brown.
3. Pour in the red wine and fresh parsley. Cover and cook for 12 minutes on high pressure. When done, release the pressure naturally and carefully remove the lid.
4. Top the steak with the butter sauce. Serve and enjoy!

Nutritional Information:

Calories 337
Carbohydrates 2.5g
Protein 34.5g
Fat 18.7g

Instant Pot Teriyaki Chicken

Prep time: 5 minutes
Cook time: 35 minutes
Serves: 4

Ingredients

- 1/2 cup soy sauce
- 1/2 cup water
- 1/2 cup brown sugar
- 2 tbsps. rice wine vinegar
- 1 tbsp. mirin (Japanese sweet wine)
- 1 tbsp. sake
- 1 tbsp. minced garlic
- 1 dash freshly cracked black pepper
- 1 lb. skinless, boneless chicken

Directions

1. Combine soy sauce, brown sugar, water, rice wine vinegar, sake, mirin, pepper, and garlic in a bowl to prepare the sauce.
2. Put chicken in an electric pressure cooker (such as Instant Pot(R)). Pour the sauce over.
3. Close lid and lock. Set to Meat function, with the timer on to 12 minutes. Give 10-15 minutes for pressure to build.
4. Gently release pressure with the quick-release method according to manufacturer's instructions, for 5 minutes. Remove lid. Insert the instant read thermometer into the middle of the chicken and make sure to reach at least 165°F (74°C). If not hot enough, cook for 2-4 more minutes.
5. Take chicken out from the cooker. Shred or cut up. Mix with sauce from the pot.

Nutritional Information:

Calories 259
Carbohydrates 33.1g
Protein 24.3g
Fats 2.3g

Teriyaki Salmon

Prep time: 15 minutes
Cook time: 5 minutes
Serves: 2

Ingredients:

- 3 tbsps. lime juice
- 2 tbsps. olive oil
- 2 tbsps. reduced-sodium teriyaki sauce
- 1 tbsp. balsamic vinegar
- 1 tbsp. Dijon mustard
- 1 tsp. garlic powder
- 6 drops hot pepper sauce
- 6 uncooked jumbo salmon

Directions

1. Mix together the all ingredients except the salmon in a big zip lock plastic bag then put in the shrimp. Seal the zip lock bag and turn to coat the salmon. Keep in the fridge for an hour and occasionally turn.
2. Drain the marinated salmon and discard marinade. Broil the salmon 4 inches from heat for 3 to 4 minutes per side or until the salmon turn pink in color.

Nutritional Information:

Calories 93
Carbohydrates 3g
Protein 13g
Fats 4g

Instant Pot Meatballs

Prep time: 5 minutes
Cook time: 30 minutes
Serves: 4

Ingredients:
- 2 pounds ground meat
- 1 small onion, finely chopped
- 4 medium garlic cloves, peeled and minced
- 2 large organic eggs
- 4 tablespoons ranch dressing
- 4 tablespoons almond flour
- 2 tablespoons fresh parsley, finely chopped
- 2 tablespoons Worcestershire sauce
- 1 cup Frank's Buffalo Hot Sauce
- ½ cup unsalted butter
- ½ cup water

Directions
1. In a large bowl, add the garlic, eggs, ground meat, onion, ranch dressing, parsley, and almond flour. Mix until well combined.
2. Preheat your broiler. Form balls from the mixture and put on a baking sheet. Broil for 10 minutes or until brown. Remove and set aside.
3. On the Instant Pot, press "Sauté" and add the butter. Once melted, stir in the hot sauce, Worcestershire sauce and water.
4. Stir in the chicken meatballs and cover. Cook for 15 minutes on high pressure. Release the pressure naturally for 10 minutes, then quick release the remaining pressure. Carefully remove the lid. Serve and enjoy!

Nutritional Information:
Calories 243
Carbohydrates 3g
Protein 19g
Fats 4g

Creamy Lamb Korma

Prep time: 5 minutes
Cook time: 35 minutes
Serves: 4

Ingredients:

- 1-pound lamb steak, cut into 1-inch pieces
- 1 tablespoon extra-virgin olive oil
- 1 medium onion, finely chopped
- 1-inch piece ginger, peeled and minced
- 6 medium garlic cloves, peeled and minced
- 2 tablespoons tomato paste
- ½ cup coconut milk or plain yogurt
- ¾ cups water
- 3 teaspoons garam masala
- ½ teaspoon turmeric powder
- 1 teaspoon smoked or regular paprika
- ½ teaspoon cardamom powder
- ¼ teaspoon sea salt
- ¼ teaspoon freshly cracked black pepper

Directions

1.   On the Instant Pot, press "Sauté" and add the olive oil. Once hot, add the chopped onions, minced garlic and minced ginger. Sauté for 1 minutes, stirring frequently.
2.   Add the tomato paste along with ¼ cup of water. Give a good stir.
3.   Stir in all the seasonings and give another good stir.
4.   Stir in the coconut milk, the remainder of the water and lamb pieces. Cover and cook for 15 minutes on high pressure. When done, release the pressure naturally and remove the lid.
5.   Serve and enjoy!

Nutritional Information:

Calories 280
Carbohydrates 5g
Protein 26g
Fat: 25g

Coconut Protein Balls

Prep time: 10 minutes
Cook time: 15 minutes
Serves: 4

Ingredients:

- ¼ cup vegan vanilla protein powder
- ¼ cup hemp seeds
- ¼ cup coconut butter
- 1 Tablespoon maple syrup
- 1 Tablespoon water
- 1 teaspoon cinnamon

Directions

1. Pulse all the ingredients in a mini chopper food processor and until combined.
2. Stir the dough and roll the mixture into small ball using your hands. You should get about 8 balls. Add some drops of water if the dough is very dry.
3. Eat immediately. You can alternatively store in an airtight container for about 4 days at room temperature or up to 2 weeks in the refrigerator or up 3 months in a freezer.

Nutritional Information:

Calories 234
Carbohydrates 5g
Protein 16g
Fats 5g

Jalapeno Turkey Tomato Bites

Prep time: 5 minutes
Cook time: 5 minutes
Serves: 2

Ingredients

- 2 tomatoes, sliced with a 3-inch thickness
- 1 cup turkey ham, chopped
- ¼ jalapeño pepper, seeded and minced
- 1/3 tbsp Dijon mustard
- ¼ cup mayonnaise
- Salt and black pepper to taste
- 1 tbsp parsley

Directions

1. Combine turkey ham, jalapeño pepper, mustard, mayonnaise, salt, and black pepper, in a bowl.
2. Arrange tomato slices in one layer on a serving platter.
3. Divide the turkey mixture between the tomato slices, garnish with parsley and serve.

Nutritional Information:

Calories 463
Carbohydrates 4g
Protein 6g
Fats 10g

Hard-Boiled Eggs Stuffed with Ricotta Cheese

Prep time: 5 minutes
Cook time: 25 minutes
Serves: 4

Ingredients

- 4 eggs
- 1 tbsp green tabasco
- 2 tbsp Greek yogurt
- 2 tbsp ricotta cheese
- Salt to taste

Directions

1.   Cover the eggs with salted water and bring to a boil over medium heat for 10 minutes. Place the eggs in an ice bath and let cool for 10 minutes. Peel and slice in half lengthwise. Scoop out the yolks to a bowl; mash with a fork.

2.   Whisk together the tabasco, Greek yogurt, ricotta cheese, mashed yolks, and salt, in a bowl. Spoon this mixture into egg white. Arrange on a serving plate to serve.

Nutritional Information:

Calories 454
Carbohydrates 8g
Protein 32g
Fats 18g

Dinner

Butternut Squash Risotto

Prep time: 10 minutes
Cook time: 15 minutes
Serves: 4

Ingredients:

- 3 tbsp butter
- 2 tbsp minced sage
- ¼ tsp black pepper, ground
- 1 tsp minced rosemary
- 1 tsp salt
- ½ cup dry sherry
- 4 cups riced cauliflower
- ½ cup butternut squash, cooked and mashed
- ½ cup parmesan cheese, grated
- ½ cup mascarpone cheese
- 1/8 tsp grated nutmeg
- 1 tsp minced garlic

Directions:

1. Melt your butter inside of a large frying pan turned to a medium level of heat.
2. Add your rosemary, your sage, and the garlic. Cook this for about one minute or until this mixture begins to become fragrant.
3. Add in the cauliflower rice, the pepper and salt and the mashed squash. Cook this for three minutes. You will know it is ready for the next step when cauliflower is starting to soften up for you.
4. Add in your sherry and cook this for an additional six minutes, or until the majority of the liquid is absorbed into the rice, or when the cauliflower is much softer.
5. Stir in the mascarpone cheese, the Parmesan cheese, as well as the nutmeg (grated).
6. Cook all of this on a medium heat level, being sure to stir it occasionally and do this until the cheese has melted and the risotto has gotten creamy. This will take around four to five minutes.
7. Taste the risotto and add more pepper and salt to season if you wish.
8. Remove your pan from the burner and garnish your risotto with more of the herbs as well as some grated parmesan.
9. Serve and enjoy

Nutritional Information:

Calories 337
Fats 25g
Carbohydrates 9g
Protein 8g

Cheesy Broccoli Soup

Prep time: 5 minutes
Cook time: 30 minutes
Serves: 6

Ingredients

- 2 pounds broccoli, chopped
- Salt to taste
- 5 cups vegetable broth
- ¼ cup shredded cheddar cheese
- 1 tbsp olive oil
- ¼ cup lemon juice
- 2 garlic cloves, mince
- 1 white onion, chopped
- Pepper to taste

Directions:

1. Heat the olive oil in a pan with medium heat.
2. Fry the onion for 1 minute and then add the garlic. Fry until the garlic becomes golden in color.
3. Toss in the broccoli and stir for 3 minutes.
4. Pour in the vegetable broth.
5. Add salt, pepper and mix well.
6. Cook for 20 minutes or until your broccoli is perfectly cooked through.
7. Take off the heat and let it cool down a bit.
8. Add to a blender, and blend it until your soup is perfectly smooth.
9. Transfer the soup into the pot again and heat it over medium heat.
10. Add lemon juice, cheddar cheese and check if it needs more seasoning.
11. Serve hot with more cheese on top.

Nutritional Information:

Calories 97
Fats 3.6 g
Carbohydrates 13.4g
Proteins 5 g

Beef Cabbage Stew

Prep time: 30 minutes
Cook time: 2 hours
Serves: 8

Ingredients

- 2 pounds beef stew meat
- 1 cube beef bouillon
- 8-ounce tomato sauce
- ¼ cup chopped celery
- 2 bay leaves
- 8-ounce plum tomatoes, chopped
- 1 1/3 cups hot chicken broth
- Salt and pepper to taste
- 1 cabbage
- 1 tsp Greek seasoning
- 4 onions, chopped

Directions:

1. Cut off the stem of the cabbage. Separate the leaves carefully. Wash well and rinse off. Set aside for now.
2. Fry the beef in a large pan over medium low heat for about 8 to 10 minutes or until you get a brown color.
3. Into the pan, pour in 1/3 of the chicken broth.
4. Add the beef bouillon, and mix well.
5. Add the black pepper, salt and mix again.
6. Add the lid and cook on medium low heat for about 1 hour.
7. Take off the heat and transfer the mix into a bowl.
8. Spread the cabbage leaves on a flat surface.
9. Fill the middle using the beef mixture. Use generous portion of filling, it will give your stew a better taste.
10. Wrap the cabbage leaves tightly. Use a kitchen thread to tie it. Finish it with the remaining leaves and filling.
11. In a pot heat the oil over fry the onion for 1 minute.
12. Add the remaining chicken broth.
13. Add in the celery and tomato sauce and cook for another 10 minutes.
14. Add the Greek seasonings, and mix well. Bring to boil and then carefully add the wrapped cabbage.
15. Cover and cook for another 10 minutes.
16. Serve hot.

Nutritional Information:

Calories 372
Fats 22.7 g
Carbohydrates 9g
Protein 31.8 g

Fried Whole Tilapia

Prep time: 10 minutes
Cook time: 25 minutes
Serves: 2

Ingredients

- 10-ounce tilapia
- 2 tbsp oil
- 5 garlic cloves, mince
- 4 large onion, chopped
- 2 tbsp red chili powder
- 1 tsp turmeric powder
- 1 tsp cumin powder
- 1 tsp coriander powder
- Salt to taste
- Black pepper to taste
- 2 tbsp soy sauce
- 2 tbsp fish sauce

Directions:

1. Take the tilapia fish and clean it well without taking off the skin. You need to fry it whole, so you have to be careful about cleaning the gut inside.
2. Cut few slits on the skin so the seasoning gets inside well.
3. Marinate the fish with fish sauce, soy sauce, red chili powder, cumin powder, turmeric powder, coriander powder, salt and pepper.
4. Coat half of the onions in the same mixture too.
5. Let them marinate for 1 hour.
6. In a skillet heat the oil. Fry the fish for 8 minutes on each side.
7. Transfer the fish into serving plate.
8. Fry the marinated onions until they become crispy.
9. Add the remaining raw onions on top and serve hot.

Nutritional Information:

Calories 368
Fats 30.1 g
Carbohydrates 9.2g
Proteins 16.6 g

African Chicken Curry

Prep time: 10 minutes
Cook time: 30 minutes
Serves: 4

Ingredients

- 1-pound whole chicken
- 1/2 onion
- 1/2 cup coconut milk
- 1/2 bay leaf
- 1-1/2 teaspoon olive oil
- 1/2 cup peeled tomatoes
- 1 teaspoon curry powder
- 1/8 teaspoon salt
- 1/2 lemon, juiced
- 1 clove garlic

Directions

1. Keep the skin of the chicken.
2. Cut your chicken into 8 pieces. It looks good when you keep the size not too small or not too big.
3. Discard the skin of the onion and garlic and mince the garlic and dice the onion.
4. Cut the tomato wedges.
5. Now in a pot add the olive oil and heat over medium heat.
6. Add the garlic and fry until it becomes brown.
7. Add the diced onion and caramelize it.
8. Add the bay leaf, and chicken pieces.
9. Fry the chicken pieces until they are golden.
10. Add the curry powder, coconut milk and salt.
11. Cover and cook for 10 minutes on high heat.
12. Lower the heat to medium low and add the lemon juice.
13. Add the tomato wedges and the coconut milk.
14. Cook for another 10 minutes.
15. Serve hot with rice or tortilla.

Nutritional Information:

Calories 354
Fats 10g
Proteins 18g
Carbohydrates 17g

Yummy Garlic Chicken Livers

Prep time: 10 minutes
Cook time: 30 minutes
Serves: 2

Ingredients

- ½ pound chicken liver
- 2 teaspoon lime juice
- 6 garlic cloves, mince
- ½ teaspoon salt
- 1 tbsp ginger garlic paste
- 1 cup diced onion
- 1 tbsp red chili powder
- 1 tsp cumin
- 1 tsp coriander powder
- Black pepper to taste
- 1 cardamom
- 2 tomatoes
- 1 cinnamon stick
- 1 bay leaf
- 4 tablespoon olive oil

Directions

1. In a large pan, heat your oil over high heat.
2. Add the garlic and fry them golden brown.
3. Add onion and fry until they become caramelized.
4. Turn the heat to medium and add the bay leaf, cinnamon stick, cardamom and toss for 30 seconds.
5. Add the ginger garlic paste and 1 tbsp water. Adding water prevents burning.
6. Add the coriander powder, black pepper, salt, cumin, and red chili powder.
7. Cover and cook for 3 minutes on low heat.
8. Add the livers and cook on medium heat for 15 minutes.
9. Add the tomatoes and cook for another 5 minutes.
10. Check the seasoning, add more salt if needed.
11. Serve hot with tortilla.

Nutritional Information:

Calories 174
Fats 9g
Protein 18g
Carbohydrates 2.4g

Healthy Chickpea Burger

Prep time: 15 minutes
Cook time: 10 minutes
Serves: 2

Ingredients:

- 1 cup chickpeas, boiled
- 1 tbsp tomato puree
- 1 tsp soy sauce
- A pinch of paprika
- A pinch of white pepper
- 1 onion, diced
- Salt to taste
- 2 lettuce leaves
- ½ cup bell pepper, sliced
- 1 tsp olive oil
- 1 avocado, sliced
- 2 Burger buns to serve

Directions:

1. Mash the chickpeas and combine with bell pepper, salt, pepper, paprika, soy sauce and tomato puree.
2. Use your hands to make patties.
3. Fry the patties golden brown with oil.
4. Assemble the burgers with lettuce, onion, avocado and enjoy.

Nutritional Information:

Calories 254
Fat 12g
Protein 9g
Carbohydrates 7.8g

Quinoa Protein Bars

Prep time: 15 minutes
Cook time: 40 minutes
Serves: 16

Ingredients:
- ½ cup almonds, chopped
- ½ cup chocolate chips
- ½ cup coconut oil, melted
- ½ cup flaxseed, ground
- ½ cup honey
- ½ tsp. salt
- 1 cup quinoa, dry
- 2 ¼ cup quick oats
- 3 large egg whites

Directions:
1. Preheat oven to 325° Fahrenheit
2. On the bottom of a clean, dry baking sheet evenly spread oats, quinoa, and almonds.
3. Bake for about 15 minutes or until lightly brown. You may want to stir the items in the cookie sheet every few minutes to ensure nothing burns.
4. Remove grains and nuts from the oven and allow to cool completely, but don't turn off the oven.
5. Whisk the egg whites in a bowl and beat the coconut oil and honey into them.
6. Combine flaxseed, chocolate chips, and salt into the cooled grains and nuts and then pour that mixture into the mixing bowl, coating everything completely.
7. Line your baking sheet with parchment paper and spread the mixture evenly onto it, pressing it into one even layer. You may want to shape the sides of the mass, depending on whether or not it reaches the edges of your baking sheet without thinning out too much.
8. Bake for 30 minutes, then remove from the oven.
9. Let cool for one hour before slicing into evenly-shaped bars, then cool completely.
10. Enjoy!

Nutritional Information:
Calories 269
Carbohydrates 30g
Fats 15g
Protein 6g

Desserts and snacks

Low-Carb Brownies

Prep time: 10 minutes
Cook time: 20 minutes
Serves: 16

Ingredients:

- 7 tablespoons Coconut oil, melted
- 6 tablespoons Plant-Based sweetener
- 1 Large egg
- 2 Egg yolk
- 1/2 tsp Mint extract
- 5 ounces Sugar-free dark chocolate
- ¼ cup Plant-based chocolate protein powder
- 1 tsp Baking soda
- ¼ tsp Sea salt
- 2 tablespoons vanilla almond milk, Unsweetened

Directions:

1. Start by preheating the oven to 350°F and then take an 8x8 inch pan and line it with parchment paper, being sure to leave some extra sticking up to use later to help you get them out of the pan after they are cooked.
2. Into a medium-sized vessel, use a hand mixer, and blend 5 Tablespoons of the coconut oil (save the rest for later), as well as the egg, Erythritol, egg yolks, and the mint extract all together for 1 minute. After this minute, the mixture will become a lighter yellow hue.
3. Take 4 oz of the chocolate and put it in a (microwave-safe) bowl, as well as with the other 2 Tablespoons of melted coconut oil.
4. Cook this chocolate and oil mixture on half power, at 30-second intervals, being sure to stir at each interval, just until the chocolate becomes melted and smooth
5. While the egg mixture is being beaten, add in the melted chocolate mixture into the egg mixture until this becomes thick and homogenous.
6. Add in your protein powder of choice, salt, baking soda, and stir until homogenous. Then, vigorously whisk your almond milk in until the batter becomes a bit smoother.
7. Finely chop the rest of your chocolate and stir these bits of chocolate into the batter you have made.
8. Spread the batter evenly into the pan you have prepared, and bake this until the edges of the batter just begin to become darker, and the center of the batter rises a little bit. You can also tell by sliding a toothpick into the middle, and when it comes out clean, it is ready. This will take approximately 20 to 21 minutes. Be sure that you do NOT over bake them!
9. Let them cool in the pan they cooked in for about 20 minutes. Then, carefully use the excess paper handles to take the brownies out of the pan and put them onto a wire cooling rack.
10. Make sure that they cool completely, and when they do, cut them, and they are ready to eat!

Nutritional Information:

Calories 107
Fats 10g
Carbohydrates 5.7g
Protein 2.5g

Apple Bread

Prep time: 10 minutes
Cook time: 20 minutes
Serves: 10

Ingredients:

- ½ cup honey
- ½ tsp. nutmeg
- ½ tsp. salt
- 1 cup applesauce, sweetened
- 1 tsp. baking soda
- 1 tsp. vanilla extract
- 2 ¼ cup whole wheat flour
- 2 large eggs
- 2 tbsp. vegetable oil
- 2 tsp. baking powder
- 2 tsp. cinnamon
- 4 cup apples, diced

Directions:

1. Preheat oven to 375° Fahrenheit and oil a loaf pan with non-stick spray or your choice of oil.
2. Beat eggs in a mixing bowl and stir until completely smooth.
3. Add the honey, oil, applesauce, cinnamon, vanilla, nutmeg, baking powder, baking soda, and salt. Whisk until completely combined and smooth.
4. Add the flour into the bowl and whisk to combine, making sure not to over-mix. Simply stir it enough to incorporate the flour.
5. Add apples to the batter and mix once more to combine.
6. Pour the batter into the loaf pan and smooth the top with your spatula.
7. Bake for 60 minutes, or until an inserted toothpick in the center comes out clean.
8. Let stand for 10 minutes, then transfer the loaf to a cooling rack to cool completely.
9. Slice into 10 pieces and serve!

Nutritional Information:

Calories 210
Carbohydrates 41g
Fats 5g
Protein 5g

Coconut Protein Balls

Prep time: 20 minutes
Cook time: 0 minutes
Serves: 27

Ingredients:

* ¼ cup dark chocolate chips
* ½ cup coconut flakes, unsweetened
* ½ cup water
* 1 ½ cup almonds, raw & unsalted
* 2 tbsp. cocoa powder, unsweetened
* 3 cup Medjool dates, pitted
* 4 scoops whey protein powder, unsweetened

Directions:

1. Blend almonds in a food processor until a flour is formed. Add the water and dates to the flour and continue to process until fully combined. You may need to stop intermittently to scrape down the sides of the bowl.
2. Add cocoa and protein to the processor and continue to process until well combined. You may need to stop intermittently to scrape down the sides of the bowl.
3. Pull the blade out of the processor (carefully!) and use your spatula to gather all of the dough in one place inside the processor container.
4. On a plate or in a large, shallow dish, spread the coconut flakes.
5. Scoop out a little bit of the dough at a time using a spoon, and roll it into balls, then roll each one in the coconut flakes.
6. Refrigerate for at least 30 min before enjoying.

Nutritional Information:

Calories 108
Carbohydrates 16g
Fats 4g
Protein 5g

Chocolate Chia Pudding

Prep time: 3 minutes
Cook time: 0 minutes
Serves: 1

Ingredients:

- ¾ cup milk, unsweetened
- 2 tsp. honey
- 1 tsp. vanilla extract
- 4 tbsp. chia seeds
- 1 tbsp. cocoa powder, unsweetened

Directions:

1. In a glass jar or container, combine all liquid ingredients and mix completely.
2. Add chia seeds and cocoa powder and mix completely.
3. Allow everything to sit for about 10 minutes before stirring once again, then sealing tightly and storing in the refrigerator overnight.
4. Stir well before eating and enjoy cold!

Nutritional Information:

Calories 329
Carbohydrates 40g
Fats 14g
Protein 14g

Blueberry Muffins

Prep time: 5 minutes
Cook time: 25 minutes
Serves: 12

Ingredients:

- ½ tsp. baking soda
- ¼ cup vegetable oil
- ¼ tsp. salt
- 1 ½ cup blueberries, frozen
- 1 cup applesauce, unsweetened
- 1 tsp. vanilla extract
- 1/3 cup honey
- 2 cup whole wheat flour
- 1 tsp. cinnamon
- 2 large eggs, beaten
- 2 tsp. baking powder

Directions:

1. Preheat oven to 350° Fahrenheit and line a muffin tin with paper liners.
2. Combine eggs, apple sauce, honey, oil, vanilla extract, cinnamon, baking soda, salt, and baking powder in a bowl. Whisk until completely combined, ensuring that there are no lumps of baking powder or soda.
3. Add flour to the batter and whisk until just combined.
4. Add blueberries and mix.
5. Fill the muffin tins and bake for 22-25 minutes or until a toothpick inserted into the middle of the middlemost muffin becomes clean.
6. Let cool for 30 minutes before transferring to a cooling rack to cool completely.
7. Serve and enjoy!

Nutritional Information:

Calories 329
Carbohydrates 40g
Fats 14g
Protein 14g

Peanut Butter Protein Bites

Prep time: 30 minutes
Cook time: 0 minutes
Serves: 25

Ingredients:

- ¼ cup flaxseed, ground
- ¼ cup honey
- ¼ tsp. salt
- 1 cup peanut butter, warmed
- 1 cup quick oats
- 2 tbsp. chocolate chips
- 4 scoops whey protein powder
- 5 tbsp. water

Directions:

1. Combine all ingredients in a mixing bowl and mix well.
2. Refrigerate the mix for 20 minutes.
3. Using a spoon or small scoop, take bits of the dough out and roll it into balls.
4. Serve!

Nutritional Information:

Calories: 107
Carbohydrates: 9g
Fat: 6g
Protein: 5g

Protein Bars

Prep time: 10 minutes
Cook time: 30 minutes
Serves: 12

Ingredients:

For the bars:

- 1/3 cup coconut oil
- 1/3 cup creamy peanut butter, unsalted
- 1/3 cup almond meal
- ½ cup milk of your choice, unsweetened
- 1 ½ cup protein powder

For the Topping:

- 2 tbsp. chocolate chips
- 1 tbsp. coconut oil
- 3 tbsp. almonds, chopped

Directions:

1. In a microwave-safe bowl, combine peanut butter, milk and all but one tablespoon of the coconut oil. Heat for 30-second intervals, stirring in between, until completely smooth.
2. Mix almond meal and protein powder into the bowl and combine well until a crumbly dough is combined.
3. Line a baking dish with a parchment paper and flatten the dough into it until an even layer is formed.
4. In a small, microwave-safe bowl, put the chocolate chips and 1 tbsp. of coconut oil and heat for 30-second intervals, while stirring in between until completely smooth.
5. Pour the mixture of chocolate over the bars and spread it evenly. Sprinkle the almonds on top and then freeze the bars for about 20 minutes, or refrigerate them for about an hour.
6. Cut into 12 evenly-shaped bars and enjoy!

Nutritional Information:

Calories 186
Carbohydrates 7g
Fat 14g
Protein 8g

Healthy Salmon Burgers

Prep time: 10 minutes
Cook time: 10 minutes
Serves: 6

Ingredients

- 2 salmon fillets
- 2 eggs
- 1/2 cup chopped onions
- 1 tbsp mayonnaise
- 1 cup gluten-free bread crumbs
- 2 tsp lemon juice
- 1/4 tsp garlic salt
- 1 tbsp chopped fresh parsley
- 3 tbsp olive oil

Directions

1. Season the salmon using salt and pepper.
2. In a skillet add ½ tbsp of oil and heat it over medium heat.
3. Fry the salmon for 2 minutes on both sides.
4. Let it cool down completely.
5. Remove them bones and mash it finely.
6. In a bowl transfer the salmon. Add the onion, garlic salt, parsley, bread crumbs, mayo and eggs.
7. Mix well and create burger patties using your hands.
8. Let it refrigerate for 30 minutes.
9. In a skillet heat the remaining oil.
10. Fry the patties golden brown.
11. Make sure to fry in batches.
12. Serve warm.

Nutritional Information:

Calories 254
Fats 20g
Protein 15g
Carbohydrates 8g

Shrimp Salad

Prep time: 15 minutes
Cook time: 0 minutes
Serves: 8

Ingredients:
- 1/3 English cucumber, diced
- ¾ cup plain yogurt
- 1 lb. shrimp, cooked & chopped
- 1 tbsp. Dijon mustard
- 1 tsp. garlic powder
- 2 tbsp. mayo
- 3 med. stalks celery, diced
- Sea salt & pepper, to taste

Directions:
1. Mix thoroughly all ingredients in a bowl.
2. Cover and put in the fridge for 15 minutes before serving.
3. Serve chilled!

Nutritional Information:
Calories 112
Carbohydrates 4g
Fat 5g
Protein 14g

Broccoli Salad

Prep time: 20 minutes
Cook time: 5 minutes
Serves: 6

Ingredients:

- ½ cup dried cranberries, unsweetened
- ½ cup pecans, chopped
- ½ cup sunflower seeds
- 1 ½ tbsp. onion powder
- 1 cup plain yogurt
- 1 lb. broccoli, chopped
- 1 small bell pepper, diced
- 1 tbsp. apple cider vinegar
- Red pepper flakes, to taste
- Sea salt & pepper, to taste

Directions:

1. In a medium bowl, thoroughly mix all ingredients..
2. Cover and refrigerate for 15 minutes before serving.
3. Serve chilled!

Nutritional Information:

Calories 234
Carbohydrates 20g
Fats 13g
Protein 9g

Southwest Chicken Salad

Prep time: 15 minutes
Cook time: 15 minutes
Serves: 8

Ingredients:
- ¼ cup extra virgin olive oil
- ¼ cup red onion, finely chopped
- 1 cup corn, drained
- 1 can low-sodium black beans, rinsed & drained
- 1 jalapeño, seeded & minced
- 1 tsp. chili powder
- 1 tsp. cumin
- 1 tsp. garlic powder
- 1 tsp. onion powder
- 2 bell peppers, diced
- 2 lg. limes, juiced
- 2 lb. chicken thighs, cooked and diced
- 2 tbsp. cilantro, finely chopped
- 3 cup quinoa, cooked
- Sea salt & black pepper, to taste

Directions:
1. In a small bowl, mix chili powder, lime juice, onion powder, garlic powder, cumin, and cilantro. Mix thoroughly and set aside.
2. In a large mixing bowl, combine all other ingredients and toss until thoroughly combined.
3. Drizzle seasoning mixture over the salad and toss to coat completely.
4. Cover and refrigerate for 30 minutes before serving.

Nutritional Information:
Calories 217
Carbohydrates 30g
Fats 9g
Protein 7g

Tuna Salad

Prep time: 15 minutes
Cook time: 0 minutes
Serves: 10

Ingredients:

- ¼ cup mayonnaise
- ¼ cup red onion, finely diced
- ¾ cup plain yogurt
- 1 clove garlic, minced
- 1 lg. stalk celery, diced
- 1 tbsp. lemon juice
- 2 small dill pickles, diced
- 24 oz. tuna packed in water, drained
- Sea salt & pepper, to taste

Directions:

1. In a medium bowl, thoroughly mix all ingredients.
2. Chill in the fridge for 12 minutes while covered before serving.
3. Serve chilled!

Nutritional Information:

Calories 152
Carbohydrates 2g
Fats 8g
Protein 18g

Greek Quinoa Salad

Prep time: 10 minutes
Cook time: 15 minutes
Serves: 6

Ingredients:

- ¼ cup red onion, finely chopped
- ½ cup feta cheese crumbles
- ½ cup parsley, finely chopped
- ½ English cucumber, chopped
- 1 cup quinoa, cooked and cooled
- 1 lemon, juiced
- 1 large bell pepper, chopped
- 1 medium tomato, diced
- 1 tbsp. cumin
- 2 tbsp. extra virgin olive oil
- 20 Kalamata olives pitted and halved
- Sea salt & pepper, to taste

Directions:

1. In a medium bowl, thoroughly mix all ingredients..
2. Cover and chill in the fridge for 15 minutes before serving.

Nutritional Information:

Calories 344
Carbohydrates 28g
Fat 23g
Protein 8g